'*Parenting in the Age of Smart Everything* is a l
raising a Gen-Alpha child. This book is a life
apart by the double-edged sword of digital med
in a dilemma between control versus freedom
book helps resolve those conflicts. It is a wel
fresh, forward-looking perspective on children's critical thinking, inclusivity and global citizenship. Both as a mom and a consumer culture academic, I found this book highly insightful and thought provoking. A must-read for parents, educators and researchers.'

Tanvi Gupta, *Faculty, Marketing Area, Indian Institute of Management Ahmedabad*

'This book will serve as a much-needed guide in parenting, especially in the context of raising Gen Alpha. *Parenting in the Age of Smart Everything* by authors Manisha Pathak-Shelat and Kiran Vinod Bhatia is a book that bridges the gap between traditional values and contemporary challenges where technology and media have silently crept into every aspect of our lives. Each chapter explores critical themes that affect the environment around the Gen Alpha and their future. It emphasises the concept of 'unlearning' that prepares all stakeholders in the school community to be more adaptable, future-ready and open to change. It further highlights the importance of cultivating tolerance to help children navigate in a fast-paced digital world. This book will serve as a much-needed guide to parents, teachers and caregivers in raising Gen Alpha with clarity, compassion and confidence.'

Malati Kalmadi, *Founder Director of the Kaveri Gifted Education and Research Centre (KGERC) and SaiSTA (Sai Skill Training Academy) and the Automotive Skilling Academy; Honorary Director at Anjali Morris Foundation*

'Pathak-Shelat and Bhatia have written a must-read analysis of digital media use among Generation Alpha. This insightful and timely book provides a critically-needed perspective on media use by young people and provides theoretically-driven strategies for both parents and educators. The authors are unafraid of tackling important issues such as negotiating diversity, promoting tolerance, and unlearning social biases.'

Karyn Riddle, *Robert Taylor Professor of Strategic Communication, School of Journalism & Mass Communication, University of Wisconsin, Madison, USA*

Parenting in the Age of Smart Everything

This book is a companion to parents in navigating the new childhood—marked by smart technology, increasing diversity, and growing uncertainties. While the Millennial and Gen Z parents of Gen Alpha are not new to technology and diversity, the speed and scale of societal and technological transformation can make parenting overwhelming. Here is a book that is more a conversation than a manual; more an empathetic guide than a bunch of thumb-rules. Parents can turn to it when grandparents can't be consulted on the new challenges and the internet throws as much misinformation as help.

The book walks parents through the challenges posed by shifting global and local dynamics, being surrounded by people who are "different" at home and at work, and the dark side of technology. The biggest contribution of the book is that it is aimed at parenting that helps children benefit from diversity and technological advances, and lead lives full of rich experiences, rather than looking at diversity and technology with fear. Additionally, the authors have proposed ways in which parents can help their children become global citizens who not only think critically, but also know how to acknowledge and negotiate their personal biases.

Showing the contribution of parenting in cultivating a growth mindset that values leadership, innovation, and responsibility, this book will be significantly useful to parents, teachers, university students, and counsellors, while offering impressive material for courses in the departments of education, child development and family studies, psychology, social work, and media studies.

Manisha Pathak-Shelat is a parent, professor, researcher, writer, speaker, and an incorrigible optimist. Manisha has a Ph.D. in Mass Communication from the University of Wisconsin–Madison, USA and a Ph.D. in Education from the Maharaja Sayajirao University of Baroda, India. She is deeply interested in understanding young people's digital cultures in all their richness and diversity. She is equally passionate about creating a world where our children find belonging, safety, and nurturance.

Kiran Vinod Bhatia is a parent, educator, and researcher at the intersection of emerging technology and next-gen users. She translates research on AI, online safety, media literacy, and global citizenship into practical routines for families and schools. An academic-turned-experience researcher, she bridges theory and practice with ease. Her passion is helping design human-centered technologies and media habits that are clear, compassionate, and actionable.

Parenting in the Age of Smart Everything

Manisha Pathak-Shelat and Kiran Vinod Bhatia

Routledge
Taylor & Francis Group
LONDON AND NEW YORK

Designed cover image: Getty Images

First published 2026
by Routledge
4 Park Square, Milton Park, Abingdon, Oxon OX14 4RN

and by Routledge
605 Third Avenue, New York, NY 10158

Routledge is an imprint of the Taylor & Francis Group, an informa business

British Library Cataloguing-in-Publication Data
A catalogue record for this book is available from the British Library

ISBN: 978-1-032-96581-9 (hbk)
ISBN: 978-1-032-96588-8 (pbk)
ISBN: 978-1-003-59004-0 (ebk)

DOI: 10.4324/9781003590040

Typeset in Sabon
by Taylor & Francis Books

Contents

Tables

Acknowledgements

It takes a village to raise a child; it turns out it also takes a village to write a book about raising children in a world that won't sit still. This project was carried out by many hands and many conversations. Our first and deepest thanks go to the parents and young people who trusted us with your stories, your worries, your experiments, your fierce hopes. You let us sit at your kitchen tables, peek into your group chats, and learn what actually helps on a Tuesday afternoon. The best lines in this book belong to you.

We are grateful to MICA for being our academic home—an anchoring place to test ideas, be challenged by students, and turn rough notes into arguments that could stand up in the light. To the mentors, early readers, and colleagues who endorsed this work and pushed us to be clearer and braver: your confidence arrived exactly when we needed it. At Routledge, Amit Kumar held faith in this project from the first page, and Srimoyee Chakraborty made the machinery of publishing feel human; thank you both for steady hands and patient guidance.

Books get finished because people show up. Debnandini Dey, thank you for your assistance in preparing the manuscript. We owe a special debt to our families for modeling the kind of parenting we write about: to Neelam Bhatia and the late Vinod Bhatia; and to the late Yogini Pathak and Chandravadan Pathak—your everyday courage, kindness, and clarity set the bar. We will carry your lessons forward.

Partnerships make both parenting and authorship possible. Julian Clark and Uday Shelat, thank you for walking beside us as co-parents and through missed deadlines and moving targets.

Revati Shelat has been our quiet compass—keeping us close to the kitchen table and away from abstractions. She has a gift for stripping a page down to the line that matters, for steering us from theory to a usable step, and for reminding us to put the phone down at dinner, listen all the way to the end, and choose presence over performance. Many of the book's most practical pages began as some gentle margin notes she shared with us in our conversations: "What if we tried…," "Say it simpler," "Show me how."

At five years old, Shane guides us in a different—and truer—way. His questions ("Why are you looking at your screen and not at me?"), negotiations about "One more minute," curiosity about robots and voice assistants, and his instinct to climb onto our shoulders have been the best training we could ask for as Gen Alpha's parents. He shows us that clarity beats lectures, choices work better than commands, repair matters more than perfection, and that play is a kind of wisdom. When our advice drifted toward adults, Shane pulled it back to the floor where the blocks are, reminding us of who this book is really for.

1 Lunchboxes and Algorithms

Consider an ordinary Tuesday morning. A parent assembles lunches; a child asks a smart speaker to convert fractions into pizza slices; a grandparent notes, not unkindly, that homework once involved pencils and paper. The device provides an answer, and life proceeds. The lack of astonishment is the signal. For today's youngest cohort—Generation Alpha—connectivity and AI are not features to be adopted; they are utilities, as unremarkable as electricity. This matters because policy, schooling, and parenting still treat "technology" as an add-on. For Gen Alpha, it is the ambient condition under which everything else operates—learning, connection, communication, play, friendship, even rest.

Gen Alpha's earliest memories have been formed through a combination of constraint and improvisation. Born from 2010 onward, many learned letters beside a parent's open laptop or met grandparents through a screen. The pandemic did not introduce technology; it normalized hybrid life. School moved between the kitchen and the classroom; pediatric care arrived via telehealth; friendships stretched across a neighborhood and a server with equal ease. The practical implication is clear: flexibility is not a perk for this generation—it is the default operating mode they expect from institutions. Rules built for single-channel instruction or nine-to-five availability will feel misaligned unless they adapt.

Their parents—largely Millennials, with older Gen Z not far behind—remember discrete waves of change: dial-up, then broadband; flip phones, then smartphones; search, then social; and, recently, AI. That mental model encourages "event" thinking: you brace for a leap, then stabilize. Gen Alpha encounters the same forces as background processes. Recommendation engines shape what appears before they choose; voice agents tutor without ceremony; generative tools turn a prompt into a draft. The resulting family tension is not primarily about values; it is about velocity and baselines. Adults look for off-switches because they recall life without them. Children differentiate "making" from "scrolling" because the feed has always been crowded, and they have grown up filtering it.

Diversity also presents differently. Millennials came of age amid campaigns for inclusion; Gen Alpha grows up inside it—and surrounded by the backlash. A single classroom may seamlessly accommodate multiple languages, new names and pronouns, and holidays from many traditions. This is not evidence

DOI: 10.4324/9781003590040-1

that identity is simple. It is evidence that pluralism has moved from statement to practice, with all the friction practice entails. The educational task, therefore, shifts: beyond celebrating difference, schools and families must teach navigational skills, how to encounter conflicting norms online and off, how to repair harm, and how to sustain one's own voice without erasing someone else's. For Generation Alpha, technology is not a field trip, but the weather—pervasive, predictable, and easy to ignore until it shifts. This reality influences the educational and parenting approaches. Beyond themed assemblies about inclusion or "digital citizenship," schools and families need to cultivate navigational competence: the ability to read environments shaped by algorithms, to evaluate sources that blur the line between news, opinion, and synthetic media, and to collaborate with AI without outsourcing judgment. In practical terms, literacy now includes understanding why a post appears, what signals steer a feed, and how an AI's confident answer can still be wrong. It also includes documenting one's own process—what tools were used, where human edits changed the output, and why—so that credit, accountability, and authorship remain visible.

Navigation also means operating across differences with skill rather than slogans. Gen Alpha encounters plural norms daily—in classrooms, group chats, and public threads—alongside debate about those norms. The goal is not unanimity; it is competent disagreement. Students need explicit coaching in audience awareness (what belongs in a private chat may not belong in a class forum), in summarizing opposing views fairly before responding, and in setting boundaries around consent for photos, tags, and reposts. Equally important is teaching repair as a civic skill: naming harm clearly, correcting or retracting misinformation, and re-entering a conversation with changed practice. These habits turn inclusion from an annual celebration into a routine of accountability and respect.

Delivering this shift does not require grand new programs, so much as disciplined implementation. Classrooms can embed quick verification rituals before sharing claims, require brief "AI use notes" on assignments, and grade for process as well as product. Families can replace blanket screen rules with purpose-specific agreements—this tool for this task, this window closed for deep work—and model consent by asking before posting about their children. Across ages, the progression is the same: start with feelings and facts, move to feed mechanics and source sense, and culminate in argumentation, disclosure, and restorative steps when mistakes occur. The outcome we should measure is not fewer screens, but stronger judgment: a generation that can read the room and the feed, speak across difference without erasing anyone, and keep human dignity at the center even when an algorithm sits at the edge of every page.

Everyday interactions with technologies are also amplified by the influx of global experiences and influences, as connection and communication become faster and more accessible. What once felt abstract now enters through the side door of daily routine. Wildfire smoke cancels recess: a conflict abroad appears as a classmate's relocation; an economic shock redraws a parent's schedule from office to hybrid to something in between. The scale is planetary; the effects are intimate. In that environment, the "basics" expand. Patience, empathy, and curiosity still matter. So do newer literacies: algorithmic awareness (how ranking and personalization work), source verification (who made this and how we know), data hygiene (what is collected, for how long, and to what end), and consent in digital spaces (what it means to share, tag, and remix respectfully). These are not niche topics anymore; they are prerequisites for safety, citizenship, and opportunity, and very much the topics of dinner table conversations.

Even before employment begins, Gen Alpha rehearses the modern workplace. Multiplayer games and group chats teach coordination across time zones; prompts to AI tutors teach specification, iteration, and error-checking; short learning loops build tolerance for feedback. The point is not to anoint children as "mini professionals." It is to recognize that the competencies adults now label as "future of work"—collaboration with tools, cross-cultural teamwork, continuous learning—are already being practiced by children on an everyday basis. The corresponding adult responsibility is governance: deciding what decisions remain human, setting norms for credit and accountability when a system assists, designing learning that strengthens judgment rather than outsourcing it, and re-centering joy and empathy in daily living.

Parenting has adjusted, if unevenly. Many Millennial caregivers, raised to prize linear achievement and visible status markers, now prioritize presence and shared judgment over blanket restrictions. The households that fare best tend to replace generic screen-time quotas with purpose-specific agreements: this tool for this task; this window closed for sustained work; this show watched together and discussed; this account private with a named adult as backup. Schools can match that posture by making tools the subject of instruction (Why did this result appear? How could the prompt be improved?), rather than the object of prohibition.

Strip away the hype, and two facts remain. First, technology has become a social environment, not a set of gadgets. It structures attention, mediates relationships, and shapes choices long before anyone notices. Second, diversity is a daily reality, not an annual theme. Classrooms, feeds, and families already reflect a wider range of identities and experiences, and the debates around them arrive early. The question for adults is not whether to permit these conditions; it is how to steward them so that human judgment, dignity, and care stay at the center.

Taken together, these dinner-table scenes and classroom habits describe more than a family vignette; they sketch the operating system of childhood now—technology as environment, diversity as daily fact, and education recast from celebration to navigation—where children learn to read the room and the feed, to argue without erasing anyone, and to repair when they get it wrong. And yet, none of this appeared overnight, which is why, before we prescribe what families and institutions should do next, we need to trace how the baseline was built—how, from 2010 to today, hybrid life became ordinary, algorithms moved from novelty to infrastructure, and global forces slipped from headlines into lunch schedules. Only by understanding that timeline can we see clearly the world Gen Alpha will inherit, and what preparation worthy of it must look like.

The World Gen Alpha Will Inherit (2010–Today)

Over the past decade and a half, the infrastructure of ordinary life has changed more than its scenery. Handheld devices have become the primary portal to information and services, instruction has shifted between physical and online formats, and personal rituals now increasingly unfold through webcams and speakerphones. What has changed isn't only the tools; it's the feeling of living inside them. Millennials and older Gen Z learned to "go online." This is true well beyond the Global North; cheaper devices and data plans have stitched more of the Global South into the same fabric, so a child in Delhi and a child in Detroit can laugh at the same clip before breakfast. And yet the kids who seem to be born with a screen in hand are often the first to test limits: classroom "minimalism" challenges, weekend phone-in-a-drawer rituals, quiet hours that reset the nervous system. They accept AI as ordinary and still ask, with growing seriousness, what kind of adults it is asking them to become—probing questions about privacy, bias, authorship, and what to do when a system's answer feels wrong but confident.

Their values formed under visible instability. Pandemic-time routines taught them how quickly the ground can shift—and how communities improvise care. Climate change doesn't live in a distant chapter, it shows up as hazy skies, flooded streets, or canceled school matches. Conflicts abroad arrive as annotated maps and first-person clips braided into the same feed as a friend's birthday video. The result is a generation unusually attuned to the ties between global events and local life; they correct a parent's recycling, fact-check an uncle's forward, and join a cause a continent away because the people who share their values sit one click from their phone home screen. Romance and family life are also carried along in the same current. While Millennials and Gen Z parents remember pushing back on scripts—dating across lines, delaying marriage, claiming the right to choose—Gen Alpha has inherited that muscle and layers onto it a wider acceptance of gender expression and identity. The paradox is that freedom can also spark a craving for steadiness: in a world that moves fast and argues loudly, some will pick old-fashioned vows and slow rituals. Whether they choose unconventional partnerships or traditional ones, they expect to own the decision—and for love to honor the lives they lead, not the ones their parents imagined.

Learning mirrors this blend of agency and flux. A new language begins with a friendly owl and a streak, rather than a workbook; a stubborn concept clicks because an educator halfway across the world framed it just right in a ten-minute YouTube video, or ChatGPT pauses without sighing and rewrites its explanation until the child at the kitchen table fully understands it and says, "Thank you, Chat!". Adults worry, sometimes rightly, about frayed attention, and kids describe a different trade: fewer hour-long trudges, more ten-minute sprints that add up, with the power to loop back whenever they like. New basics slip in alongside literacy and numeracy: algorithmic awareness (why did I see this?), source sense (who made it and how do I know?), and co-writing with

AI (when to use it, when to put it away). Even their mental picture of work tilts with these habits. Instead of a single ladder, they imagine a set of bridges and teams scattered across time zones. "Success" stretches to include time, health, impact, and the ability to say no. Standing in the middle of it is AI: co-writer, lab partner, friend, tutor, counselor, analyst, and synthesizer. The question isn't whether AI is in the room, but about the role it should play and how to keep human judgment, care, and creativity in charge.

Threads: Technology, Learning, Everyday Life

Classrooms are no longer insulated from the tools that shape the rest of daily life, and the central question is not whether students should use AI, but how they should use it. The appropriate stance is neither alarm nor uncritical embrace; it is supervised collaboration that treats the system as fast but fallible and insists on human judgment as the final step. That requires explicit routines: disclose when a model was used, specify the prompt and the intended purpose, compare the output to trusted sources, and revise in public view so that authorship remains visible. This is literacy for the present tense, and it belongs in every subject, rather than in a single "digital citizenship" unit. Parents will need this literacy as much as the kids.

Pluralism has likewise moved from poster to practice. Families will have to learn how to welcome friends from diverse backgrounds and to sensitively discuss with their kids if there are any reservations or concerns about their children's friendships. Schools and families must teach competent disagreement and repair: summarize an opposing view accurately before critiquing it, separate people from claims, ask permission before posting photos, and correct rather than quietly delete when a mistake circulates. These are not etiquette tips; they are civic skills that reduce harm, build trust, and keep public spaces usable.

Economic reality enters early as well. Children see remote work reshape family schedules, as they see older siblings and parents stitch together income from creative gigs that combine manual work and machine assistance. Many parents will have their professional identities shift several times while their children are growing up. The lesson should not be that all jobs are precarious or that every task will be automated. The lesson is that success will rely on a blend of durable capacities—clear communication, self-management, ethical use of tools—and a willingness to learn across changing roles. "What do you want to be?" is a smaller question than "What problems do you want to work on, with whom, and under what constraints?". Schools can help by assessing process and reasoning, not just outcomes, and by insisting that human judgment, credit, and accountability remain legible when systems contribute.

None of this is simple, but it does not need to be theatrical. It asks parents and teachers to admit uncertainty, to model verification, and to design rituals that hold even as tools change—phones in a basket at dinner, walks after hard days, weekends with family and friends, a standing rule that big questions can interrupt small tasks. If we want children who can live well inside the hum of the present, we must give them practice in the skills that make communities work: humility when the system is confident and wrong, curiosity when difference is real and nearby, and repair when harm occurs.

Hybrid school schedules, algorithmic feeds, and global events all converge at home, where choices are daily. Kitchens and bedrooms turn abstractions into routines: bedtimes, homework, and group chats become the settings where habits form. Families teach privacy and consent through concrete steps: ask before posting a photo, limit location sharing, and review settings together. Multigenerational households operate in inclusion, with simple practices such as using stated names and pronouns, and recognizing multiple holidays. The world reaches children through many channels, but home routines determine how they respond and what they retain.

The Home They Grow In: Parenting, Tensions, and Bridges

If Gen Alpha moves differently, it's also because their parents are parenting differently. Many Millennial caregivers were raised by Boomers or Gen Xers who prized stability, linear achievement, and visible markers of status—top marks, prestigious degrees, secure jobs. In places like India, the first glow of economic liberalization cast a bright sheen on material success and the dream of studying or working abroad; social media arrived later, as an adult accessory, rather than a childhood environment. Today's parents toggle between wanting to protect children from screens, and wanting to equip kids to use them well. They refresh parenting threads for tips more often than they call their own parents, try to make up for moments their jobs once stole, and watch digital footprints with a mix of vigilance and fatigue. When work allows, they push for balance not as a luxury, but as a strategy for showing up—for dinner, for bedtime, for the messy middle of homework. Labels like "Boomer," "Gen X," or "Millennial" never capture the full global picture, but across contexts you can feel the same pivot from performance to presence, from rigid rules to shared judgment.

Different childhoods behind you and different futures ahead of you mean friction is part of the deal—and the house tends to heat up in predictable ways. Identity and inclusion are one of the brightest spark-points. Gen Alpha is the most diverse cohort many schools and neighborhoods have ever seen; they treat difference as the default, expect classmates to be called what they want to be called, and want libraries, holidays, and heroes to mirror the mix of their lives. Parents who grew up with diversity as an aspiration sometimes feel caught between pride and discomfort when the conversation turns sharp—about sustainability choices, about who gets represented and how, about a joke that lands wrong. Screens and attention form another fault line: a parent sees "more time online," a child insists they're "making, not just scrolling," and both are a little right. Autonomy and risk round out the trio: kids push to try, test, and post, while parents brace for harms they've read about and sometimes lived. What helps here is naming the shared aim out loud and returning to it when the room gets tense. The goal is to return to a place in conversation where dignity isn't theoretical, but mandated for both children and parents. From that shared aim, families can practice the small moves, such as listening first, asking "Show me how you're using it," explaining the why behind a boundary, revisiting decisions after a trial period—small and novel steps that turn friction into fuel for understanding.

The final truth is humbler and more hopeful than any rulebook: no recent cohort of parents has had to admit so openly how uncertain they feel about what "future-ready" even means. Norms that once felt solid now wobble, and advice that worked yesterday ages fast. Work becomes less about predicting the path and more about learning to walk it together, testing, adjusting, learning, repeating, so that both generations can keep their footing on moving ground. In that spirit, this chapter lingers where families actually come together: at the kitchen table where a math problem meets a voice assistant, in the car ride where pronouns and policies get sorted out in real time, at a birthday celebration where different world views of the extended family members collide, in the quiet after lights-out when a child wonders what tomorrow's world will ask of them. The more we understand the world Gen Alpha is growing up in, the better we can help them build it.

A Quiet Promise for What's Next

Every night, as our apartment quiets and the morning's frustrations have been replaced by bath time negotiations, after-dinner treats, bedtime discussions, and the ritual of choosing tomorrow's socks, my child asks a question that lands with both feet in the future: "Will the robot be my boss?" A hundred possible answers crowd the doorway. I often take the path I've been practicing all day, the one this chapter has tried to trace: "Sometimes the robot will help. Sometimes it'll be wrong. Our job is to know the difference—and to decide what kind of people we want to be while we're deciding." It's a small sentence with a big promise tucked inside: we don't control the current, but we do control how we travel together.

If there is a single throughline to carry forward, it is that Gen Alpha's world is less a set of gadgets or slogans, and more a cyborgian biome—technology as environment, diversity as daily reality—into which old human questions have been moved. How do we learn? With whom do we belong? What is our work for? Those questions age well. They invite the same virtues across eras—patience, empathy, courage—even as the tools and terms change. The discussion above has lingered in classrooms and kitchens not because they are quaint, but because they are where big forces touch small lives, and where the practices that matter—asking, noticing, choosing with care—are trained.

For parents and educators, the task ahead is not to predict a path that refuses to hold still. It is to build ways of walking: routines that keep bodies and relationships at the center; agreements that translate values into concrete choices; shared language that lets a five year-old and a tired adult talk about privacy, authorship, and rest without turning every conversation into a test or argument. It is to treat friction as information, not failure—to ask what a conflict is trying to teach, adjust, and try again. It is to remember that "future-ready" is a posture, not a checklist: a blend of discernment ("Is this true?"), agency ("What can I do about it?"), and solidarity ("Who can I do it with?"). And amidst all this, retain the joy and spontaneity that define childhood!

So, we end up as we began, in a kitchen that could be anywhere. A lunchbox lid shuts. A backpack zips. It will still be about a grandparent telling a story about a map that used to live in a glove compartment, and the child holding up a phone that contains all the maps, from everywhere, all at once. The argument worth having, the one that will repeat in larger and more different forms as our children grow, is not only "How do we get someplace?", but "What do we want the trip to feel like?"

The chapters that follow encourage us to keep asking and answering that question, so that the everyday noise of their world becomes less a source of anxiety and more a dial we can adjust—until it works as a fit place for growing up.

2 Negotiating Diversity

Stranger Danger—or Stranger-Savvy?

How real is "stranger danger" in 2025? The phrase was minted for a world without group chats, rideshares, or video doorbells. Our kids live in neighborhoods where the doorbell is a camera, the playground rules are posted by QR code, and the "stranger" might be the gamer they've built a castle with for six months, but never met in-person. Parenting inside that reality is thrilling and exhausting. We want children to grow into confident, kind people in a society that feels safe and fair. Then the news cycle floods our feeds with violence, hate crimes, scams, and abuse, and our instincts narrow: trust the inner circle, side-eye everyone else. Clothing, language, food, prayer—difference itself can start to read as risk.

Here is the tension this chapter tackles: shutting down is not the same as staying safe. Generation Alpha is growing up in families and communities that don't fit yesterday's template—single-parent and blended households, same-sex parents, multigenerational homes, foster and adoptive constellations, immigrant and multilingual communities. Their classrooms and group chats are diverse by default. The task, then, isn't to warn them away from every unfamiliar person or place; it's to help them become stranger-savvy. That means practical skills they can use anywhere: reading context, setting boundaries, naming discomfort, and getting help—offline and online. It means learning digital street smarts too: recognizing manipulative DMs, spotting AI-generated fakes, using privacy controls, and knowing when to leave a thread. It also means noticing green flags, not only red ones: adults who introduce themselves clearly, spaces with visible rules and check-ins, peers who accept "no" without pressure.

We won't pretend every encounter is safe. Recognizing risk signals—offers of secrecy, urgent pressure, gifts tied to favors, requests to move to a more private channel—is a survival skill. But blanket paranoia steals too much, such as new friendships, joyful cultural exchanges, helpful neighbors, and mentors who change life. This book aims to help parents and teachers raise children who are both open-hearted and alert—kids who can speak up against cruelty and bias, who can negotiate differences with respect, and

DOI: 10.4324/9781003590040-2

who can protect their own well-being without shrinking their world. We will show how fear can be amplified by feeds and neighborhood apps, how suspicion can harden into bias, and how communities slide from cautious to toxic. We will also show how to reverse that slide with routines any family or school can adopt: clear consent practices, check-in plans, code words, buddy systems, disclosure about AI use, and scripts for "No," "I need to ask my grown-up," and "I don't keep secrets that make me uncomfortable."

Before we dive into the mechanics—how children learn who they are and where they belong through family stories, media diets, and school culture—let's take a quick temperature check. Think of it as a warm-up for your real muscles and your empathy muscles alike. Grab a pen and try a short "Stranger-Savvy" quiz: a few recent, real-to-life scenarios from playgrounds, DMs, carpools, and team chats. Your answers will give you a baseline, and the rest of the chapter will give you tools to tune that baseline—less fear, more skill, and a wider, safer world for our kids.

Quiz Time

Do your children have friends who are from different religious communities?

1 No. I don't think it is advisable to allow young children to befriend people who have a different religion. They might get influenced.
2 No. Children are gullible and if they are exposed to different beliefs, they might want to leave our religion.
3 Yes. I have always encouraged my children to meet new people and experience different lifestyles.

What are your views on refugee children?

1 They should have an equal chance of finding success in personal and professional life.
2 They should be willing to serve the hosts in low-level roles.
3 They should accept the fact that young people from the host country will find more success in life.

Do you share your utensils with the house helps in your homes?

1 No. House helps are not clean, given the nature of their jobs, and so we can't allow them to eat and drink from the same utensils.
2 We have separate utensils for everyone in the house, including the house helps.
3 Yes. Why should we have separately marked utensils for them?

Do you often use religious, racial, or caste- and class-related slurs in your families?

1 Sometimes. I try not to use them in front of the children, but sometimes my tongue slips.
2 I don't use them in front of my children, but these words are a part of my vocabulary.
3 Never. I am not comfortable using these words at all.

How often do you accept your mistakes in front of your children and apologize for your mistakes?

1 I don't think I should apologize as a parent.
2 I don't apologize or accept my mistakes, but I try to make up for it in a different way
3 I always apologize and ask for forgiveness

What do you think about the new regulation that poor children should be admitted to all schools. Would you be happy for your child to have these children as friends?

1 I wouldn't be very excited. Children who belong to different backgrounds won't be able to mingle well.
2 I am comfortable if the school accepts children from a lower economic background. I will not, however, allow my children to befriend them after school hours.
3 Yes. I would like my children to be exposed to different realities and family backgrounds.

Once you have marked your answers, calculate your total score using the serial number of the options selected as the value of your response. Write down this score on a separate piece of paper and keep it safe.

Becoming a critical and conscious adult is a lifelong process. The term "parent" or "teacher," we believe, is a verb and not a noun. It isn't something you did. It is something that you continuously engage in and work on. We are always in the "process of being a parent," which means we must consciously evaluate and improve our methods of nurturing children. Regardless of how you did in the quiz, this book will help you critically examine your engagement with children and draw from a wide array of resources to improve your style and pedagogy.

Mirroring the Adults

The results of the quiz give you some idea about your worldview and how you look at those who are different. There is a high chance that either your worldview will influence your children, or you will enter into conflict because they do not accept your treatment of strangers.

Does the following conversation ring a familiar bell?

MAYA: (coming home while her mother hosts guests) That new kid, Amir, is so unfair. He didn't pick me up for handball, and I had to sit out the whole class. If I'm ever captain, I'll make sure kids like him don't get to run the game.

RINA: (Mother): (sharply, glancing at the guests) Mind your words. Is that how you speak in front of people?

MAYA: (puzzled) What did I say? You always call him "the boy from somewhere else" and say we shouldn't get too close. And "unfair" isn't even bad. You say worse things about the families who just moved here.

RINA: (embarrassed) Enough. Go wash up. I'll serve lunch.

MAYA: (heading to her room) So it's fine when you say it, but when I repeat it, everyone acts shocked.

Children are keen observers. They consciously and subconsciously model behavior of the adults around them—their actions, words, thought processes, and emotions. During the formative years of a child's development, adults, especially parents and family members, act as a bridge, linking children with the world outside. Adults initiate children into everyday activities, belief systems, values, codes of conduct, and ethics, thus helping children understand how they should behave in relation to people, places, and communities.

This is part of the process of socialization, i.e., the process through which children are trained to play their role in the world. Children learn who they are as they take up social roles in their lives. For instance, children brought up in religious families begin to engage with the concept of "God" from an early age and are trained to perform actions which articulate their relationship with God. They participate in religious rituals, perform certain rites, and develop a particular lifestyle, influencing their food preferences, clothing choices, and other everyday activities. These everyday practices help them cultivate opinions about the world, and religion becomes one of the lenses through which they look at themselves and others. The process of socialization, thus, is multilayered and very complex. It broadly operates at three levels:

1 Individual: At this level, children learn about their social roles and the accepted modes of performing these within families and societies. For instance, children may adopt several social roles, such as that of a religious person, a student, a family member, a citizen, a friend, and so on. As they learn how to behave from within the boundaries of these roles, they look for examples in adults around them, and perceive them as role models. They study their parents' behavior, for instance, to identify socially acceptable ways to perform each of these roles within their communities. Observing adults in their surroundings helps them understand how they should define themselves: Who are they? Are they Hindus/Muslims/

Christians? Others? Are they seen as rich or poor? What is their gender, and how should they act like a girl/boy? What are their family, social, and educational responsibilities and expectations? It is through socialization that children develop a notion of the "self."

2 Others: This notion of self is defined in relation to others in society. For instance, if a child performs her role as a daughter, she regulates her behavior in relation to parents or grandparents in the family. Right from a young age, children are taught what they can do, watch, feel, and say in accordance with the norms and rules normalized within societies.

   Being a girl, they might impose certain limitations on her, and there will be certain expectations too. In some families, she may be required to help her mother in the kitchen, as her brother and father sit in the drawing room playing board games or watching TV. Similarly, her brother will learn that performing his role as the boy translates into not participating in household chores, but taking care of supposedly more manly tasks, such as heavy lifting, taking care of repairs, or running certain errands, and expecting his sister to manage the kitchen and the house. As is evident, the brother and sister have learnt how to situate themselves in relation to the other gender. The problem begins when this creates hierarchies in society, labeling one role as superior and the other as inferior. This applies to class, caste, and religious differences as well.

3 Community: Each community creates a set of rules, regulations, and norms to ensure that individuals behave in ways that reinforce the authority of their community. These communities are a local network of family, friends, professionals, neighbors, and acquaintances who belong to the same social groups based on class, caste, religion, gender, and so on. For example, specific church denominations, caste associations, women's associations, or clubs. Children interact with many such communities from a young age and learn how to abide by the rules and norms created by their communities. Also, parents often refer to these community expectations while socializing with their children within set societal norms.

Based on their observations of how the adults in their lives behave, children learn to internalize biases toward others, practice hatred against individuals who have a different lifestyle, and design violent ways of punishing, abusing, and reprimanding those who challenge their worldviews, faiths, and beliefs.

To be honest, accepting something that is "different" is not always easy. We are often suspicious of other people who look different, have a novel lifestyle or culture, or just a different way of seeing the world. Realizing that parents, teachers, family members, and other adults are responsible for sowing seeds of biases and prejudice in the minds of young people can be unsettling, especially when we love them and care for them. As a result, most of us refuse to evaluate our stake in the process of raising children who are biased, intolerant, and scared of interacting with people who are not like themselves. Also, many of us are unaware of our own biases toward other individuals, belief systems, practices, and processes.

Additionally, many parents would prefer their children to accept the family's worldview without friction. That expectation, however, is harder to sustain with Generation Alpha. Constant exposure to peers, platforms, and algorithms gives them access to perspectives that often diverge from what they hear at home. As a result, questions and disagreements are not outliers; they are the predictable outcome of a wider information diet and a broader social sphere. At the same time, adults are not simply resistant to change; they are responsible for safety. Headlines about online grooming, harassment, and real-world harm make supervision feel prudent, not punitive. Parents and teachers may wish to grant full freedom across online and offline spaces, yet the risks they fear are not imagined. The result is a persistent tension: young people push for autonomy informed by many sources, while adults set boundaries informed by a duty of care. This is not a failure of either side. It is a normal feature of intergenerational life that calls for clear rules, shared judgment, and ongoing dialogue.

How to Address Our Fear of Strangers

We often guard our children from diverse interactions because we have learnt to associate strangers with danger! But "different" doesn't always mean bad or evil, superior or inferior. In the chapters that follow, we also talk about real risks and how to recognize and deal with them while broadening the social circles of our families. We also acknowledge that sometimes differences are painful, and we cannot always embrace or accept them. Some communities and groups have difficult histories to grapple with. At other times, we feel that the rules of the game are not the same for all the players. In such situations, we must find ways to be tolerant and, at times, advocate for our beliefs and lifestyle in order to stand by our values. We will talk about these tensions in later chapters.

Is the Difference Always Inferior?

Across the world, discrimination based on social identities is deep-rooted and complex. We not only avoid people who are different, however, rather the tendency is to label them as inferior, discriminate against them, abuse them, and, in extreme cases, enact violence towards them. This is damaging our social fabric and making many people miserable. For peace and development in our society, we need to raise children who can happily navigate and enjoy a diverse and multicultural society, while knowing and respecting their own roots and cultures. For this, it is first important to understand how children develop a worldview, i.e., how they cultivate opinions about other individuals and the ways in which they learn how to engage with different people in their societies. There are three major institutions in society that socialize children—family, school, and media. Examining how these institutions influence and shape our children's worldview will help us identify new ways of raising our children, such that they grow into individuals who are prepared to ask important questions, enact compassion, and work toward establishing social justice in their societies.

The Big Three: How Family, School, and Media Shape Our Children

Family, school, and media are the three most important building blocks constituting children's worldview. While families and schools allow children to learn and practice norms and codes of conduct acceptable to the communities and countries where they live, the media are a channel that connects children's local environments, as well as the outside world. Children's perception of how power and politics work in the world, their meaning-making of things not experienced firsthand, their mental images of people and places, and their perception of their own place in the world are largely influenced by the media.

Let us look at one example. Young girls learn about gender roles that are dominant in their immediate communities through family members, teachers, friends, and peers through routine interactions. Several cultures see a slim body as a desirable quality in women, and a muscular body for men. Similarly, many families and communities in South Asia, for instance, want their girls to be fair-skinned because only fair skin is considered beautiful. Fair becomes synonymous with lovely. In many schools, the fair girls are often cast as female protagonists in theater activities and other school programs, such as cultural dance performances, video making, and so on.

The obsession with fair skin is instilled among children by their families and communities through everyday communication and practices. It gradually also translates into discrimination against dark-skinned people, considering them less valuable. This obsession over fair skin is then reinforced through media narratives where celebrities endorse beauty products designed to make girls look fair and lovely. The media act as a bridge between children's local experiences and the trends and practices dominant in the outside world. It is, however, important to realize that the popular culture in the outside world and everyday experiences in their immediate surroundings are not mutually exclusive or hierarchical. They happen simultaneously and constantly feed each other. It is also possible that these girls are exposed to media that question discrimination based on body type or skin color. Now they have exposure to a different set of opinions and values that question what they have received from their families. For Gen Alpha, because of their exposure to the world beyond their geographic boundaries, such questioning is common.

Children are socialized based on an interaction between what they observe and practice at home, schools, and communities, and how these patterns of thoughts and actions are normalized and justified in and through media and popular culture. What is significant in this spiral of socialization is the interdependence of these two worlds. Let us look at how the three building blocks which constitute children's worldview—families, schools, and media—function within this interaction between the macro (larger) and micro (at an intimate level) forces of socialization.

Home: Observing, Learning, Practicing

Homes can be considered rich learning sites where children are introduced to four crucial social identities: religion, gender, caste or race, and class. Let us look at the following example:

Scene: A Playdate Refused

Azad, twelve, stands in the hallway with his backpack half-zipped. "Can I go to Mateo's after school on Friday? We're finishing our science project and then his mom said we can play a video game. He lives three streets away. I can text you when I get there."

His mother, Beli, does not look up from the cutting board. "We don't know that family," she says. "They're new. Different churches, different customs. And these days, you can't be too careful. Invite him here instead—when your father is home."

Azad tries again. "We know them a little. Mateo's mom came to parents' night. She's a nurse. Our teacher paired us. Their building has security."

Beli's mother calls from the dining room. "Son, stay with your own. We don't eat outside. People cook differently. What if they make you something you shouldn't have? What if they take you somewhere? The news is full of stories."

Azad's sister, Tia, looks up from her homework. "He went to Neil's' house last week without any of these questions," she says quietly.

"That's different," Beli replies. "We have known Neil's family for years. This is not about being unkind; it is about safety. Text Mateo and say you can't go. Tell him we have plans."

Azad types, then pauses. "What should I say?"

"Say we don't do playdates at other people's houses," grandmother answers. "It's our rule."

He sends the message. The hallway is suddenly very quiet.

What the Child Learns

Nothing openly hateful was said. Yet a clear lesson was delivered: unfamiliar identity equals elevated risk; "stranger danger" applies not only to unknown adults in public spaces, but to classmates whose faith, language, food, or country of origin differ from the family's own. Safety language did the work of boundary-making. The mother invoked news headlines and "not knowing them" to justify a blanket ban. The grandmother added cultural and dietary cautions that, in practice, functioned as a proxy for race and religion. The rule appeared neutral—we don't do playdates at other people's houses—but it was applied inconsistently, enforced for some families and not for others. The sibling noticed the double standard. The boy absorbed it.

This is how fear is socialized at home. A reasonable aim is to keep a child safe, but it becomes a categorical policy that narrows a child's world and codes difference as danger. The immediate effects are small but consequential. A science partner becomes "the new boy we don't visit." A text full of enthusiasm turns into a polite refusal. A budding friendship loses momentum. At school the next day, when Mateo asks why, Azad will reach for the language he heard: "We don't go to other people's houses. My mom says it's not safe." The message lands twice—once on a friend who now understands he has been placed outside the circle, and once inside Azad, who has practiced equating unfamiliarity with risk, rather than practicing how to assess and manage risk.

Over time, these home policies scale. Children who are repeatedly told to "stay with your own" learn to avoid mixed groups, to decline invitations, and to interpret cultural difference as a warning sign, rather than a green flag to learn. They miss chances to build cross-cultural fluency, to negotiate consent and boundaries in new settings, and to identify genuine safety markers (clear introductions, reachable adults, agreed pickup times, visible house rules). They also miss the more ordinary goods of childhood: a new game, a different lunch, a friend's family story. The intention was protection. The outcome is a narrower map of who counts as safe and a weaker set of navigational skills for the diverse world the child already inhabits.

Schools: A Social Playground

Schools can be defined as a social playground where children learn social behavior, relations, attitudes, and values. There are three reasons why schools are so instrumental in children's development as responsible adults and members of society:

1. In school, children learn through peer interactions, which is a very powerful means of training children as members of a social community. Many studies argue that children are more receptive to certain attitudes, values, and behavior when they observe their peers perform these in social settings. Schools provide a fertile site for these peer interactions to unfold.
2. In the formative years, teachers are one of the strongest influences, and children model their behavior either to imitate the teachers or to please them. In either case, teachers encourage their students to perform certain social behaviors which they deem important. Sometimes, these social behaviors may reinforce gender, religious, caste, and class biases in classrooms and normalize stereotypes prevalent in society.
3. Children spend most of their time in schools in many countries where school timings extend for seven to eight hours per day. As a result, the experiences children have in school influence them in significant ways. Also, schools can be considered proxy sites for children to experience the outside world. Children bring to the classroom their family socialization, social identities, beliefs, and values. These diverse realities and identities interact with each other in classrooms. Children's engagement with these interactions informs their attitudes and beliefs toward those who have different lifestyle practices. It is, therefore, crucial to identify classrooms as places where children experience differences prevailing in societies for the first time; classrooms are also the place where children can learn critical skills required to live with these differences.

As is evident, children's socialization is braided with their school experiences. If the school reinforces their learnings from home about stranger danger, they are encouraged to see all those who are different as dangerous. If the school trains them to challenge this learning and encourages diversity, there is an initial conflict in a child's mind. In this case, the school must be sensitive enough to help the child resolve this conflict.

Media: Constructing Social Realities

Media—both legacy media such as television, cinema, and newspapers, and digital and internet-based media—act as a lens through which children witness and participate in the outside world. The media perform two critical functions in socializing children. First, the media inform and influence the aspirations of children in relation to how they should position themselves in their societies. Second, the media legitimize several social identities prevalent in society and encourage the audience to practice these identities in and through these everyday interactions. For instance, young children who have been raised on the staple diet of item numbers in Hindi commercial cinema often sing, dance, and appreciate these songs in their routines. We observe that many child contestants on children's talent shows are encouraged to dance seductively on racy and adult songs in order to become more popular and get more votes. Repeated and continuous exposure to such TV content normalizes the act of sexualizing children's bodies and encourages children to look at themselves using the same lens. Similarly, if they routinely experience a stereotypical and biased representation of a community or a social identity in their media exposure, they normalize that representation as the whole truth and the only truth about that identity.

It is important to note that the role of the media is not limited to just representing society as it is. Media not only select issues that should trend or be covered in the mainstream, but also encourage individuals to understand these issues in limited, particular ways. For instance, youth who are fans of Hollywood Westerns would be encouraged to perceive the indigenous people in a narrow, antagonistic manner unless they are exposed to counter-images by other media sources. Even in Bollywood, different regional communities are represented in a derogatory manner to get laughs, e.g., Gujaratis are business-minded, and Sikhs lack intellect. If not encouraged to think critically, the young audience would easily consider these portrayals to be reality.

As is evident, this limits the meanings people associate with a phenomenon, community, event, and/or experience. For instance, several scholars have critiqued the role of media in granting space only to fringe, radical, and violent voices while discussing issues related to religious conflicts in India. In each religious community, we find people who are working hard to initiate interfaith dialogue and to establish peace between different communal factions in the country. These voices are never heard on prime-time news channels, for instance, because voicing moderate opinions doesn't help them garner more

TRPs. On the other hand, sensationalizing issues of public concern, especially those related to religious differences among communities in India, helps news channels sustain and/or increase their viewership and the revenue earned from advertisements, sponsorships, partnerships, and other forms of economic and political alliances. When children, as well as adults, consume a media diet that essentially sensationalizes the differences between religious communities, individuals start believing that their religion will ultimately decide their fate in the world. Constant exposure to and consumption of such media stories can influence children's everyday interactions with those from different religious communities.

It is difficult for children to imagine forms of conduct different from those normalized by their families/communities and reinforced in and through media. Though media have the potential to present new possibilities and to enable individuals to reimagine ways of being in the world, most capitalist media ventures do not like to make people feel uncomfortable. They provide content that aligns with the dominant thoughts, practices, and values in society. When children consume media uncritically, instead of questioning the content based on principles of equality and justice, they reproduce the aspirations and lifestyle choices projected by the media in their routines. This is how the media socialize children to behave within religious, gender, class, and caste norms.

As we just discussed, families, schools, and media are the three core dimensions in children's socialization as social entities. Recognizing these three dimensions as crucial sites where children learn most of their social behavior is the starting point toward designing critical and inclusive experiences for them, so that they can thrive in a diverse and multicultural world.

Adults can pay close attention to their personal biases as they educate and bring up children. This, we believe, entails the massive project of "unlearning." Adults must be open to the idea of unlearning certain beliefs, values, attitudes, and practices if they intend to ensure that their children/students are equipped with the critical skills required to question the standards of behavior normalized in our society.

In the next chapter, we elaborate on how adults can unlearn their biases to create a healthy and inclusive learning environment for their children.

3 Learning to Unlearn

The Unlearning Process

Unlearning is the most difficult kind of learning. Unlearning involves re-examining our daily habits, beliefs, and practices; our inherited and acquired baggage. It can be as simple as the husband taking equal responsibility for chores and emotional labor in the family, to something as complicated as expanding and enriching your social circles to meet people who are from a different social background. For instance, it can be very difficult for individuals who have been raised to maintain caste or racial boundaries to introduce changes in their families by inviting people from a different caste or race to their homes. Also, such changes can have serious consequences. For instance, if an upper caste family in India decides to befriend people from the lower caste and invite them to family gatherings and celebrations, such as wedding ceremonies and so on, they might face resistance from the other upper caste relatives and guests. This can jeopardize their social relations and may compel them to retract their steps. Similarly, people who have only lived in small towns with religious and racial homogeneity would find it difficult to accept immigrants in their close social circle. Now think of major steps, such as marrying a person from a different religion or accepting your child's gay or lesbian identity. The question then is twofold: How can adults identify and unlearn social biases inherent in their thinking and practice?; and How can adults redesign their social environments to be as bias-free as possible?

To answer these questions, we have designed a step-by-step guide based on research by several scholars who work in the area of raising children in diverse and pluralist societies. Let's walk through the four-step process.

Step I: Acknowledge

The first step toward identifying personal biases is to acknowledge that our worldview needs to be constantly modified in order to keep pace with the changing times. Every worldview is incomplete, and until we acknowledge this, we cannot change our engagement with the world around us. If we constantly nourish our thinking with fresh ideas and experiences, we can easily spot gaps

DOI: 10.4324/9781003590040-3

and faults in our understanding. This aspiration to evolve into better, more sensitive, and critical individuals must emanate from within us. Unless a person truly wants to change and grow, no one else can initiate them into this process of self-discovery through unlearning. Our children can be of great help in recognizing the areas where we need to change.

Step II: Confront

Once we have acknowledged the need to constantly engage with new ideas and perspectives, it is then important to confront our own biases and to challenge them. Confronting personal biases can be difficult because, as individuals, we are socialized to believe that true faith requires unquestioning submission. As a result, we grow to consider our faith, values, and practices as sacrosanct. Also, they provide us with a solid comfort zone. This critical task of questioning oneself can put individuals in a state of "existential crisis" when and if they realize that the values and worldviews they had been holding onto are necessarily flawed. For instance, after raising two beautiful daughters with all the love and care the father can offer, if he is confronted with a reality check by one of his daughters who claims that his decisions related to their upbringing were extremely patriarchal and violated their rights, he can feel lost. It is, therefore, important to appreciate such moments of dissatisfaction and resistance every day and, as they surface, to identify the gaps, flaws, and faults in our understanding as adults.

Confronting these flaws in ourselves is a nerve-wracking process, but it can prove to be extremely beneficial for the health of the family and society. We suggest two strategies to help adults practice accepting the fault lines in their thinking. First, we should always be ready to apologize to our children if we are wrong. This helps them realize that individual growth is not a linear process. Even when you are an adult, you are still open to learning new things, making mistakes, and working toward improving yourself. It will also help children understand that learning and unlearning are processes that operate simultaneously. We cannot learn new things without unlearning our old biases. Second, include children in discussions and ask them for their opinions. Ask them, "How do you feel about this?". In India and several other countries, children are raised conventionally as "dependents" who have no say in important matters related to the house or society. This is changing, but still quite prevalent. This is wrong because, in doing this, we take away their voices from them. We steal from them their ability to ask questions related to issues that impact them. Most importantly, we take away from them their right to participate in the process of growth and development. Children must be encouraged to express themselves because they are new learners who are not uncompromisingly influenced by the social biases prevalent in their societies. Listening to our children can help us gain alternative ways of looking at people and the world.

Step III: Reimagine

Reimagining ways of being in the world can be very difficult. How can we step beyond our socialization as adults and reimagine lifestyle choices that support equality and peace? Reimagining requires that we step out of our comfort zones, deploy new analytical lenses to evaluate our practices and values, and, based on this self-introspection, experiment with unexplored ways of engaging with the world. For instance, Gen Alpha will be working in a much more sexually diverse environment than any other generation. In the beginning, parents might find it difficult to accept several different genders in place of the conventional binaries of women and men. And if they strongly influence their children's views on gender, their children might also find it difficult to work on gender-diverse teams.

Parents can start by modeling the reimagining they hope to see. Do a short self-audit of language at home and retire casual labels or jokes about "other" people; replace them with names, roles, and facts. Learn the basic vocabulary of gender and inclusion from credible guides, then practice it out loud so it becomes natural, using a person's stated name, asking for pronunciation, offering your pronouns when appropriate, and correcting yourself without drama if you slip. Diversify the family's media and bookshelf, so children regularly encounter protagonists and professionals across genders, cultures, faiths, and abilities. Write a simple family charter that makes values visible: we use people's stated names, we ask before posting photos, we don't share private information, we don't use slurs, and when we get it wrong, we repair it. Build small routines that turn values into muscle memory: a weekly "pause–ask–check" moment about something new a child noticed; a monthly "one new place, one new person" experiment, such as visiting a community center event or hosting a mixed-background playdate; a quick role-play where you practice how to respond if someone misgenders a teammate or makes a stereotype in a chat.

Then widen the circle so your child can practice inclusion with real stakes and support. Seek extracurriculars that assemble mixed teams—robotics, theater, debate, community sports—where collaboration outruns similarity, and rotate hosting so your home becomes a safe, supervised hub for diverse friendships. Partner with the school: ask how names and pronouns are recorded, how shared spaces are made welcoming, how bullying is reported and repaired, and whether teachers receive ongoing training on AI literacy and inclusion. When conflict inevitably arises, focus on repair, not punishment: guide your child to name the harm, make a visible correction, and set a plan to prevent repeats. Offer scripts they can use—"Please don't share that photo," "Let's check a source," "I'm stepping out of this chat"—and back them up when they use these. Track progress like any other skill: once a month, ask what you tried, what felt hard, and what you'll try next. Reimagining is not a one-time leap; it is a series of small, consistent experiments that expand a child's competence and, at the same time, their compassion.

Coming back to our present lives, we still learn gender-based discrimination between boys and girls at home, in schools, and through media. For instance, though cooking and household chores are crucial and valuable functions in society, they are still considered only a woman's domain in cultures across the world. Girls should have access to a larger set of experiential learning activities that broaden their horizons and their thinking related to who they can be when they grow up. Similarly, it is equally important to include toys and gaming experiences that encourage our sons to perceive activities related to managing homes and families as critical roles for the healthy functioning of society. For example, boys should be encouraged to own and use kitchen sets, get interested in cooking and cleaning the house, and perform tasks that compel them to develop sensitivity and express emotions. This is a helpful way for them to understand other genders better.

In this case, for instance, reimagining requires infusing old leisure practices of children with innovative play options that help them challenge the dictates of gendered norms and behaviors. Girls must be equipped with a sense of confidence, necessary to believe that it is possible to take up all diverse roles and professions. At the same time, they should also be made sensitive to the pressures, demands, and challenges of the world of work that men routinely experience as "providers." When boys are taught to "man up" and act invulnerable, we deny them the opportunity to seek solace and guidance in the healing powers of articulating their struggles to others through interpersonal exchanges. Also, research shows that men who believe in gender equality are less prone to violence.

Step IV: Implement

This is the most complex and formidable part of the unlearning process. How do we implement new, reimagined ways of being in the world? How do we negotiate the resistance and questions posed by members of our communities? How do we address the risk of social exclusion and threats concomitant with this process of progressive change? How do we comfort ourselves when we worry that the new choices may make us or our children more vulnerable to risks?

A three-pronged approach has worked well for many, and you may want to try it. To begin with, initiate changes in your lifestyle and home gradually and casually. For instance, instead of accusing your family and community members of being casteist or racist, initiate dialogues related to the violence embedded in such practices of exclusion and discrimination. An interesting way to do this is by sharing a news article or a video as a starting point for a discussion in the family's living room, and also encouraging children to introduce you to such media. Using the living room for this discussion is important because we want our children to know more about the inequalities existing in society and, as a family, to devise ways to address them. When children are involved in these discussions, they believe that they have a stake in this process, as they encounter realities governed by caste, race, gender, class, religion, and other social identities every day. They may also contribute interesting observations to the discussion, and we should encourage that.

The next step is to create safe spaces for children and other family/community members to narrate their stories of experienced discrimination, especially when the family identifies as belonging to a community that is marginalized in a society. They may consume movies with a storyline that shows discrimination, or they may witness instances in which they feel excluded from group activities in schools because of various aspects of their identities. If your family's language, caste, race, or regional origin is different from the dominant groups in any place, your children might feel isolated or excluded. In all such instances, we can equip our children with skills and values to make sense of the hostility they face in the world. In doing this, however, we must be careful not to create a sense of fear and hatred in the minds of young children, and not to force them into gender, religious, caste, race, or class silos. It helps to look beyond binaries such as us–them, good–evil, and God–demon. Most of the time, we all experience discrimination, and we also participate in discriminating against others. It helps to generate critical stories consisting of the varied nuances existing in society in order to discuss how different communities engage with each other, how our histories mold us, and how we are powerful in some situations and powerless in others. This includes admitting the faults in one's community, while highlighting moments of hope which exist in the form of individuals and groups in other communities who are progressively working toward creating inclusive societies. We are so hardwired to define ourselves in binaries and constant conflict with others—"I am a Muslim (who is against Hindus)," "I am a boy (who is never supposed to act like a girl)," "I am fair (which is more acceptable than dark people)"—that it becomes hard to visualize how our identities and experiences are layered and often overlap with those who are pushed to the other end of the spectrum. This is not to say that our differences are not real or that even if you find something in a group, community, or gender difficult to accept, you must unquestioningly accept it as good. We might not be able to accept certain practices, even when we are open to change.

Unlearning is required to be able to create constructive dialogues, practices, and social movements for peaceful co-existence. This begins at home and in schools, where children can acknowledge their experiences of suffering and pain. This, we believe, is the work of intimacy in families and schools.

Practicing What We Preach

Children are quick to spot if there is only preaching and no practice. It is very easy for children to ignore or reject the principles we preach if they fail to see us practice those values in our everyday lives. Practicing principles of social justice and equality is a challenging task because it is accompanied by risks of social exclusion or ostracization. For instance, it can be very difficult for parents from an extremely conservative and patriarchal family to justify their son's actions of becoming a painter or opting for a specialization in Family and

Community Sciences, largely because these fields are considered feminine, with low earning potential. Parents and grandparents may be used to a linear career path, which Gen Z and Gen Alpha are now questioning. Unconventional choices are braided with moments of internal tension, friction with others, and a lot of self-doubt. To ease this transition from self-doubt to self-change, we list some easy guidelines:

1. Study your routine behaviors at home and in schools, and identify practices that need to be changed. Table 3.1 is a snippet of the "Change Wishlist" created by one of the parents we worked with closely. It will help our readers design similar templates for themselves. We can use this template to list everyday practices where we can introduce changes in order to break gender, religious, caste, class, and other social biases.
2. Be careful of the words you use in front of your children. Many adults don't realize that using religious, caste, race, class, and gender slurs in the presence of children normalizes the practice of using a particular community and gender as a site to enact violence. For instance, when parents use forms of gender abuse that refer to sexuality or sex organs (for example, referring to the vagina), they normalize the idea that women's body can be used as a site to construct and enact violence. Similarly, when adults in the family use casteist, racial, and classist slurs, and other similar forms of abuse, they are uncritically denigrating certain castes, races, and classes at home and in schools. This can encourage children to repeat these words and internalize negative bias against other individuals and communities.
3. Involve other family and community members in this process, so that the resistance and threats from individuals of the in-group can be minimized. The most effective way of encouraging other adults to be a part of this process is by inviting them to events and experiences where guests of different genders are invited, or events curated to promote interfaith/caste/race/class dialogues. Another way of leveraging the support of your community is by sympathizing with their inhibitions to change. Community and family members who think differently should be addressed as "team members," and not as "opponents". There are many reasons why they think the way they do. It doesn't help to label them as racist, misogynistic, or bigoted without understanding and addressing these reasons.

> We can use the following phrases while engaging with those from our in-groups who resist our proposition to discard discriminatory ideas and practices: I understand, I can sympathize, let us think through this together, let us revisit some of the scriptures/texts together, and most importantly, we can't justify violence/discrimination.

Table 3.1 My change wishlist

	Unlearn	*Reimagine*
1.	I allow my sons to stay out for work or with friends till late, but my daughter is expected to be home by 7 pm.	The same rules should apply to sons and daughters. If I am concerned about the safety of my daughter, I will provide either extra resources or support to ensure that she can stay out till late without facing any problem. For this, I might have to put in more effort, such as arranged drop-off and pickup, but I am prepared to do that.
2.	I don't allow my house helps to eat and drink from the same utensils because they belong to a lower caste.	I will have to unlearn my biases that people from a lower caste are unclean. My household help ensures that my house is clean. Instead of trivializing her role in our home, I will try to normalize a humane and sensitive relationship with her.
3.	I don't allow my children to frequent the houses of their classmates who are from a different religious community.	I will acquaint myself with the families of my children's classmates who belong to a different community, and try to establish a relationship of acceptance and trust with them. In doing so, I will be more willing to allow my children to experience a different culture and/or lifestyle.
4.	In our house, only the mother cooks and takes care of the children. Every time the father is requested to help with the kids, he makes excuses and refuses to participate.	If both parents are working, we will divide household chores and contribute equally. If only the father is working, he will volunteer to help share the emotional labor of engaging children during weekdays, while contributing toward household chores during his days off from work.
5.	I don't like it when my children play with children from lower economic backgrounds in the community parks and other spaces. I, therefore, frequent only my society's parks and gardens with my children.	This practice will instill in them a sense of contempt for the less privileged people and make them incapable of understanding how economic inequalities impact people in our societies. I will, therefore, change this practice and encourage my children to frequent spaces accessed by children from diverse economic backgrounds.

Raising children in such fractious times is a special kind of calling. It is like cultivating hope and investing a sense of joy and gratitude in our children, so that they may be prepared to navigate through hatred without succumbing to the pressures of conforming to social norms.

4 Learning and Teaching Tolerance

A Huge Challenge

The World Today: Intolerance, Conflict, Violence

We began researching global citizenship more than a decade ago. We found many people around the world who identified as global citizens, and we were hopeful that in the decade to follow, many more would. These global citizens were individuals who loved their countries and cultures, and took pride in them. They weren't rootless individuals, but rather members of close networks, with strong family and community ties. While they had rich and meaningful local lives, these global citizens connected, through heart and mind, with those who were geographically distant. However, when we look around, watch the news, or scroll down our social media feed today, we see increasing signs of conflict and unrest all around us. Suddenly, diversity, inclusion, and equity are seen as negative words—words to be banned or ridiculed. It is so scary and disheartening at times that we even start questioning if it makes sense to discuss diversity and tolerance anymore. Religion, race, and class have always been the dividing factors that were used to justify discrimination and violence, but now newer factors, such as language and ethnic histories, have been added to the list for creating conflict. But then we talk to the children and young people around us, look into their hopeful eyes, witness their aspirations and dreams—this is when we strongly feel that we cannot give up and absolve ourselves of all responsibilities for the world we are shaping for Generation Alpha.

Our field visits have taken us to different cities and towns of India—from the small villages of Telav and Ghuma in Gujarat, to the sprawling cities of Delhi and Mumbai. We have both traveled to many countries of the world. All our visits have led us to believe that the virtue of tolerance and compassion has saved us from destruction. Even when periods of invasion and violence disrupted the harmony of our society, and when discriminatory beliefs and practices threatened the well-being of vulnerable groups, there have always been attempts by thinkers, leaders, artists, and many ordinary citizens to restore peaceful co-existence.

These observations help restore our hope that we can still shape the workplaces, cities, and villages we love to call our homes through the practices of respecting diversity, tolerance, and co-existence. Given a choice, we would all

DOI: 10.4324/9781003590040-4

want our children to live in places where they are safe and can thrive, no matter what their gender, caste, or religion is. Well, we can build such places only if we contribute to maintaining the harmony of our societies. For that, some leaders advocate celebrating and embracing difference, while some advise accepting difference, and if we cannot bring ourselves to do either of these, the least we can do is practice tolerance.

Many scholars have questioned the use of the word "tolerance," implying that tolerance may or may not include acceptance. The phrase "I tolerate them" has a negative connotation because here, the word "tolerate" is spoken as an obligation toward the laws/rules of the country or society. For instance, when we use the phrase "We tolerate people from other cultures," we articulate a sense of compulsion, rather than acceptance. We, however, wish to argue that this is a rather narrow and colloquially generated meaning of the word. The noun tolerance encompasses much more than the act of "tolerating the other." Tolerance is a process of creating a space for the most uncomfortable, divergent, or radically different ideas to thrive. Tolerance is an ideal wedded to practices of compassion that allow people to experience sympathy toward those who are very different from us. Tolerance involves accepting the faults in our thinking and the discontinuities in our understanding of the world. To be tolerant is to start from a place of self-doubt and acknowledge that whatever we think and/or believe is only a partial approximation of the truth. At the very least, however, tolerance is not attacking others, physically or emotionally, because they think and behave differently from us. At the very least, tolerance also involves putting up with some discomfort.

Intolerance begins with small things, and it is also not that simple to differentiate between personal preferences or likes, and dislikes and deeper values.

Pause and Think...

Suppose you are living in a township with a multinational business. You are vegetarian and find the smell of fish cooking disgusting. Naturally, the presence of a neighbor who cooks fish every day is bound to cause genuine unease. Suppose you hate dogs and are also allergic, but in your township, some people treat their dogs like their children—it is "If you want to love me, you have to love my dog." Suppose you have been raised in a strictly heterosexual ideology, and you find it difficult to accept gay couples. Your nephew has a partner who is a man, and the couple is present at several family functions. What rights do you have to preserve your way of life and preferences, and when do you have to let go to respect others? For this one difference or some discomfort, would you shut them off and keep them away completely? Worse, given a chance, would you attack them verbally or physically?

In the following sections, we explain why the practice of tolerance is critical for the health of both democracy and the rich diversity of cultures. We discuss why it is important to raise Gen Alpha with values of diversity, inclusion, compassion, and tolerance. We also draw from world leaders who, time and again, have reminded us to follow peaceful co-existence, even with our very real differences.

Tolerance is Amiable Co-Existence

Unlike what many people think, tolerance is not indifference toward others or a refusal to engage with them. In the world of today, with long histories of travel, migration, and intermingling of people, can we imagine any community living in complete isolation? Are the regressive and mythical ideas of purity, pollution, and fear of contamination from other cultures supported? Every day, each one of us enters multiple transactions at schools, offices, streets, public spaces, entertainment sites, and so on. Our children go to school and have the opportunity to befriend others who have different belief systems and lifestyles. Similarly, at work, we have colleagues from diverse social backgrounds who bring new perspectives and insights into our office spaces. We learn about people, projects, and places that speak to the diversity inherent in our culture and societies.

Ideas of purity and pollution draw strength from a belief that we can reach or possess an absolute truth; they are nested in a refusal to question the partiality of our own beliefs and opinions. This condition to proclaim one's truth as absolute is the cause of intolerance in our societies.

Let's take the example of religion. For a devout, practicing Christian, this process may involve asking questions related to the inbuilt oppression in the act of proselytizing to the masses—a phenomenon which was witnessed by many previously colonized countries in the Indian subcontinent, in Africa, China, Japan, and elsewhere. The colonial project was designed around the religious doctrine of proselytization and led to mass violence and oppression. The historicity of our colonial past weighs heavily on our present, as we think about the many Western imports that turned religion into a public spectacle and a tool for dividing the populace. Similarly, as religious individuals, Hindus should be willing to denounce the oppressive practices of the caste system and create just and more inclusive ways of organizing in their communities. Conservative Muslims need to ask why anyone who refuses to accept Islam as the only true religion should be labeled a kafir and should be a target of hate. What is more interesting is that even within every religion, there are so many ways of making "us and them" boundaries—Catholics and Protestants, Shaivaits and Vaishnavaits, Shia and Sunnis! And then there are atheists who ridicule everyone else, while everyone else looks at them with suspicion!

Once we get into the habit of creating walls, it is never-ending.

Tolerance in Practice

According to world leaders such as Gandhi, Nelson Mandela, the Dalai Lama, and Martin Luther King, among others, tolerance is a civic virtue that compels people to meet their opinions, religious beliefs, political ideology, and everyday practices with extremely seasoned skepticism. The differences in our societies can be in tension without being at war with each other. Tolerance, in our contemporary societies, can be defined as IDEA:

- Identifying the historical roots of the prevailing difference.
- Defining common goals, and shared interests and aspirations.
- Eliminating violent impulses and substituting them with participatory and democratic practices rooted in ideals of justice and empathy.
- Acknowledging tensions in our societies due to unassimilable differences, and negotiating with them through public dialogue, deliberation, and debates.

Pluralist countries and societies like India will always be home to people with several different beliefs on every aspect of life. These beliefs will sometimes appear to be irrational, and yet people are sentimental and emotional about them. Conflicts arise when these irrational cultural and religious beliefs clash with progressive civic goals. For instance, a riverside city moves to enforce clean-water rules during a major festival by restricting plaster-of-Paris idols painted with chemical dyes, and by directing immersions to lined tanks. Many devotees view river immersion as non-negotiable and see the curb as an attack on their faith. They may also respond with stronger resistance if they feel that such practices are not questioned in regard to celebrations by other religions. Municipal officials frame the policy as a public-health and environmental measure tied to potable water, fish kills, and sewage loads. The clash is immediate: neighborhood committees organize protests and vendors resist switching materials, while resident groups cite water-quality targets and court orders. Here, a belief that feels sacred to practitioners collides with civic goals—safe drinking water, ecological protection, and equal river access—illustrating how sentiment and regulation can pull in opposite directions unless regulations are introduced fairly and dialogue produces workable alternatives (eco-friendly clay, natural dyes, scheduled immersions, and designated ponds). Similarly, animal sacrifices may have been part of certain religious practices, but that should not stop us from examining it from the point of view of non-violence and animal rights.

People will continue to hold some of these beliefs or rituals, but it is important to establish the private–public distinction, so that people do not establish their own beliefs as societal standards and enforce others to adopt and practice them. Tolerance is learning the boundaries of the public–private, and while we may continue to perform certain rituals in our homes and personal lives, the public should be governed and regulated according to the consensus. In the following section, we will look at some examples of co-existence and consensus-building.

Philosophies and Traditions: Lessons in Co-Existence

The Indian subcontinent has produced competing philosophies, ideologies, and practices, and signals a tradition in a synthetic approach. According to this approach, new ideas are continuously added to the existing system of thought, without trivializing the existing or old ideas. Let's look at the story of the arrival of the Zoroastrian community in India.

> Sometime in the 10th century, a small group of Parsees, or the Zoroastrians, fled execution in Persia and reached a port in Gujarat. When they petitioned King Jadav to provide them refuge in Gujarat, the King expressed concern over the assimilation of these foreigners in India. He demonstrated this concern by showing the guests a bowl full of milk to the rim. To address this concern, the four Dasturs, i.e., elders, from the Parsee community requested a spoon of sugar. One of the Dasturs put the spoon of sugar in the milk, stirred it, and remarked that the Parsee community will become a part of the local culture, just as sugar dissolves in milk. Though they will retain their sweetness, i.e., their distinct qualities and faith practices, they will adapt to the local culture and add sweetness to it. The local Gujarati populations accepted them as their own and to this day, they have stayed true to their promise and become an integral part of India.

Like the Zoroastrians, many other communities traveled far and wide, and found refuge in the Indian subcontinent. Similarly, people from the Indian subcontinent have traveled to other countries, and have contributed richly to their host cultures.

Many spiritual traditions in the Indian subcontinent emphasize the need to co-exist and practice peace and tolerance in our thoughts and actions. Kabir's writing has influenced generations of people with profound messages on co-existence in a simple colloquial language. In Gujarat, the poets Akho and Narsinh Mehta combined social critique with spiritual messages. Bauls are wandering village singers from Bengal who have no images, temples, scriptures, or ceremonials. In their songs, they critique social divisions in our societies based on caste, class, and religion, while propagating a syncretic religious sect that combines lyrics from both the Hindu Bhakti movement and the Sufi traditions that seek to usher in humanism and empathy as bedrocks of a tolerant and pluralist society. Most of the Baul songs illustrate a beautiful synergy between Hindu and Muslim traditions, and normalize the power of a tolerant society where people with differences can co-exist.

Similar to the Baul singers are poets, artists, and saints of the Bhakti movement in the Indian subcontinent who aimed to bridge the chasm between Hindus and Muslims, upper and lower castes or Dalits, between different regional cultures, and between sexes. The Bhakti movement promoted the religion of love, tolerance, and compassion as a bedrock of an emancipated society. It was an anguished but peaceful protest against the orthodox, casteist, or classist societal traditions, by promoting common participation, shared goals, and making spiritual spaces and experiences accessible to everyone. The Bhakti movement was strengthened by the work of Sufi saints and peers who challenged Islamic orthodoxy, and combined

Vedanta philosophy and Buddhism in an attempt to question the Islamic doctrine of one truth and one God. Sufi saints preached about love and tolerance, and were highly revered across several faith communities. These verses appealed to the universal emotions and morals of love and compassion, and were also referred to in Adi-Granth, a Sikh religious text. This intertextuality, i.e., adopting ideas from other religions, resonates with the practice of tolerance, wherein traditions are evaluated for their benefit to the common goal of humanity, and all the principles, teachings, or actions that further this goal are accepted unanimously.

In the Buddhist philosophy, tolerance is equated with the presence of an awakened heart-bodhichitta, a heart that feels the pain of others regardless of social, religious, and class differences. It emphasizes the need to go beyond our interests, motives, and beliefs to feel compassion toward others.

Like Buddhism, Jain traditions also stress that training in tolerance and non-violence is indispensable. Jainism encourages people to combine multiple perspectives, several partial truths, and the many valid representations (*anekantavada*), while interacting with others and their surroundings. Many contemporary Jain monks are re-interpreting Jain philosophical traditions to address the needs of an increasingly globalized and plural world.

Practicing Tolerance: Challenges and Questions

Tolerance unsettles us. Getting out of our comfortable and familiar zones, and letting go of the certainty, is indeed not easy. We live in very fragile times where things are changing rapidly. The birth of India is tied to the story of bloodshed during partition, and it continues to tarnish Hindu–Muslim relations. Similarly, many countries of the world have been born out of violent struggles with their colonizers, and the scars of the past years are still observed. These collective memories of hatred and power struggles raise the question: How do we move into a new world and leave this baggage behind? How do we practice tolerance and negotiate differences in our lives every day? We have found some helpful lessons from the discipline of communication. These lessons help us in our daily interactions with our children and others, and also inculcate good communication skills in our children.

The Words We Use

We often use words casually, without giving full attention to their implied meaning or the effect they would have on someone. Reality is constituted through language—the words we use to describe our relationship with others. Words give us the power to connect with others or to build walls. With our words, we can either attain a state of oneness, or make visible the existing crevices of hatred in our intercommunity relations (see Table 4.1).

How can we enter a new world through communication that builds bridges rather than creates walls? While engaging in a conversation, we should pay attention to three things: what we are doing; why we are doing it; and what

Table 4.1 Inclusive alternatives to divisive words

Divisive word/phrase	*Why it can divide*	*Inclusive alternative*	*Example in sentence*
"You people/Those people"	Othering; lumps individuals into an out-group	"People in that group," or name the group specifically	"People in the after-school program raised this concern."
"Real Americans/Indians/etc."	Implies some citizens belong less	"Fellow Americans/Indians," "community members"	"Fellow Americans are split on this issue."
"Illegal alien/illegals"	Dehumanizing; criminalizes identity	"Undocumented immigrant/person"	"Undocumented students need clear guidance."
"Third world/underdeveloped"	Outdated, pejorative	"Global South," "low- and middle-income countries (LMICs)", "majority countries"	"Partnerships with LMICs improved vaccine access."
"Minorities" (as a blanket)	Vague; can erase local majorities	"Underrepresented groups," or name groups	"We're recruiting from underrepresented groups in STEM."
"Foreigners"	Othering in diverse societies	"International visitors," "newcomers," "immigrants"	"Our city welcomes newcomers through this program."
"Normal" vs. "not normal"	Centers one group as the standard	"Typical," "common," "less common," or name specifics	"This is a less common learning style."
"Boys will be boys"	Excuses harmful behavior	"Everyone is responsible for their actions"	"Everyone is responsible for treating classmates with respect."
"Man up/Grow a pair"	Polices gender; shames emotion	"You've got this," "Let's try a brave next step"	"Take a breath—you've got this."
"Act like a lady"	Polices girls' bodies/behavior	"Please be respectful," "Please sit safely"	"Please be respectful while others are present."
"Bossy" (for girls)	Penalizes leadership in girls	"Assertive," "Take the lead," with feedback on tone	"You took the lead—let's make sure everyone's heard."
"That's so gay"	Uses identity as insult	"That's not okay/unfair/confusing"	"That policy is unfair to new students."

Divisive word/phrase	*Why it can divide*	*Inclusive alternative*	*Example in sentence*
"Crazy/insane" (as a synonym for bad)	Stigmatizes mental illness	"Confusing," "overwhelming," "risky," "harmful"	"That deadline is unrealistic."
"OCD about it"	Trivializes a disorder	"Particular," "detail-oriented"	"She's very detail-oriented about formatting."
"Addict/junkie"	Reduces person to condition	"Person with a substance use disorder"	"We offer support to people with substance use disorders."
"Committed suicide"	Criminalizing language	"Died by suicide"	"We lost a teammate who died by suicide."
"Wheelchair-bound"	Implies limitation only	"Wheelchair user"	"Our venue is accessible for wheelchair users."
"Colored people"	Outdated, offensive in many contexts	"People of color," or name the community	"We're partnering with Black entrepreneurs."
"Non-white"	Defines by lack	"People of color," or name the group	"Support for Asian American founders increased."
"Transgenders" (as a noun)	Incorrect, othering	"Transgender people," "trans people"	"Transgender people face higher barriers to housing."
"Both genders"	Erases nonbinary people	"All genders"	"Restrooms are available for all genders."
"Preferred pronouns"	Suggests optional	"Pronouns"	"Please share your name and pronouns."
"Housewife" (as default)	Limits roles; gendered	"Stay-at-home parent," "full-time caregiver"	"He's a full-time caregiver this year."
"Maid/servant"	Classist; demeaning	"Household worker," "domestic worker"	"Household workers have the right to contracts."
"Master/slave" (tech terms)	Violent historical connotations	"Primary/replica," "leader/follower"	"Use a primary/replica database setup."

Divisive word/phrase	*Why it can divide*	*Inclusive alternative*	*Example in sentence*
"Blacklist/whitelist"	Links color to bad/good	"Blocklist/allowlist"	"Add these domains to the allowlist."
"Ghetto" (as an adjective)	Classist, racialized	"Low-quality," "makeshift," "budget"	"This is a makeshift solution for now."
"Gypped" (slur)	Ethnic slur (anti-Roma)	"Ripped off," "cheated"	"We were cheated by that vendor."
"Powwow/tribe" (casual use)	Appropriates Indigenous terms	"Huddle," "team," "community"	"Let's huddle after the meeting."
"Spirit animal" (casual use)	Appropriative of sacred practices	"Role model," "I relate to…"	"She's my role model in public speaking."
"Culture fit" (hiring)	Masks bias; favors sameness	"Values alignment," "job-relevant skills"	"We're hiring for values alignment and skills."
"Low-skilled workers"	Demeaning; ignores expertise	"Entry-level," "essential workers," "roles not requiring a degree"	"Essential workers kept services running."
"Language barrier"	Frames multilingualism as a problem	"Language access," "language difference"	"We'll provide language access support."
"You speak good English"	Backhanded; implies outsider	"How many languages do you speak?" or avoid comment	"Would you like materials in another language?"

would happen once we have done it. Thinking about the outcomes continuously is useful in choosing words that unite us, rather than divide us.

This does not mean that we will have no differences. We will always have differences. Communication offers both hope to dissolve the difference, if possible, but also an acceptance that some differences are unassimilable. Maybe we can create a new space altogether—a third, more cosmopolitan space, where the differences do not capture our entire attention, as we look for new realities and identities. Like any new practice, it might be difficult in the beginning. It will never be a cakewalk, especially when parties involved in the process are learning it at a different pace. It is a disorienting practice when the rug of certainty must be pulled from beneath our feet as we step into new conversations. However, these new conversations help people forgive their past trauma and conflicts. They encourage them to imagine a better future, despite the seemingly irresolvable differences in our present, and to hold on to the last ounce of compassion and understanding, as we create bridges and undo boundaries. We will encounter fear, uncertainties, backlash, and ridicule in the process.

Resolving Conflicts: Talking Through our Differences

As we discussed earlier, most of us prefer to remain confined to our echo chambers and befriend those who support our views and opinions. Well, it is the easier path, if not interesting or enriching. It is like the difference between sticking to an expressway and taking a more scenic route. Most of us do not actively seek out people with different ideologies, and initiate discussions and conversations with them. We don't encourage our children to do so either, or if they are adventurous, we are quick to reprimand them, fearing for their safety. Despite our efforts to avoid confronting differences, more often than not, the real changes we witness in our societies have been possible only when people made efforts to engage with those who were on the other side of the ideological spectrum. For instance, one of the most powerful reasons why India is less homophobic today than it was some ten years ago is that people from the LGBTQIA community strived to create spaces where they could convey and express their experiences and ideas. When these ideas reach people who either did not understand or chose not to engage with the idea of homosexuality, there is a possibility of change, even if slowly and grudgingly.

Why Conversations Are Important

We have to come together in conversations. The relationship between people and their communities is conversational. The aim of conversations is not necessarily to agree. A good conversation creates possibilities of navigating messy situations and conflicts without practicing aggression, hate, or violence. With regard to resolving conflicts, any conversation should have three core elements:

- First, the language of care, wherein we indicate a sense of respect for all the conversationalists, and ensure that each has an equal stake in the speaking–listening process.
- Second, the tone of comfort is such that everyone feels included and heard.
- Third, sensitive content signals a deep empathy for the experiences and realities of others.

Unlike terms such as debates and discussions, the term conversations is, in a sense, personal. It involves an equilibrium between the people involved, as each person articulates their narratives and stories. Personalizing conversations related to conflicts can initiate in people a sense of connection with and responsibility toward others. For instance, instead of discussing the problem of Islamophobia, if we turn toward the personal stories of our Muslim friend, Fatima, our response to the narratives of lived discrimination will be more sympathetic and kinder. Similarly, if we listen to the anguish of our Hindu friend, Avinash, as a global minority, when most of the world is divided between Islamic and Christian blocs, we understand his insecurity. An impromptu conversation with a stranger on the riverbank in Budapest, watching the line of shoes reminding us of the gruesome killing of Jews, opens our eyes to the centuries of violence they have endured. Our heart breaks when we hear firsthand our friend, Anita, talking about how difficult it was to come out as a woman, when her entire family wanted her to stay as Anil, a male identity he was assigned at birth. Conversations lay open the many ways in which these conflicts affect not some abstract notion of a specific community with a label, but people we know—our friends, teachers, co-workers, and neighbors. Also, when we try to learn about others through conversations, we are willing to learn unique and novel things about them, which will challenge the existing stereotypes. For a Muslim woman who was raised to believe that Hindus are violent and intolerant, conversations can be a great starting point to learn otherwise. Her interactions with Hindu women at her workplace may reveal that there are differences within the Hindu community—some people are conservative and would choose not to associate with Muslims, while others may be warm and welcoming; some are vegetarians, while others devour biryani and kebabs. It leads to the realization that no community is a monolith, and there are many internal differences and novelty.

It is quite likely that we might have a personal negative experience with an individual of another religion, race, or nationality. The question is, how sensible is it to transfer this limited experience to the entire group of that community?

Framing: What Are You Looking At?

Here, framing plays a very critical role. A frame is like a window through which we look at a picture. If our window is wider, we take in more of the scene. Similarly, if we include historical narratives, present realities, and future possibilities in our conversations, it allows for more space and complexity. For instance, in conversations with members from the ST/SC/OBC community on the quota system in India, if we consider how they have suffered systemic discrimination and marginalization, and how the high caste privileges have been putting generations of others in an unfair situation in (public) life, we will find it easier to understand their demands to use and hold onto the reservation system in the country. At the same time, we will also be able to see how some members of the creamy layer of such groups take unfair advantage of the system and may damage the chances of other poor people.

Conversations are not so much about persuasion, as about "thinking through together." Conversations should ideally help people raise important questions and arrive at conclusions that most effectively speak to their realities and emotions. We can have a perfectly harmonious relationship with people who have different views and ideologies.

To understand how this is possible, let's draw an example from one of the episodes of an English original show. In this episode, three schoolboys—a gay English kid, a Muslim kid, and a white English kid—are best friends. The Muslim kid invites his other two friends to his birthday party and promises that he will inform his parents that one of his friends is gay. At the party, however, he reveals that he has not been able to gather the courage to tell his Muslim parents that he has a gay friend, to which the gay friend refuses to enter the house and stands at the gate. When the father comes to the door to resolve the issue, he invites the gay kid to the party, even though his religion teaches him otherwise. The father explains that his faith is very important to him, and even though he goes to the mosque regularly, he cannot claim he understands everything. The one thing he knows for sure is that the gay kid is his child's best friend, and so he is welcome in the house.

The Muslim father, in this case, chose to hold on to his belief without qualifying his interpretation or morality for others. Many people may criticize this approach as relativism, but we interpret it as a method of sitting with differences without translating them into acts of unkindness or hate. What the father did was accept that his religion teaches him that homosexuality is wrong, but he will not practice it by being unkind and cruel to someone else.

It is natural to feel apprehensions, such as, Will I, in the process, lose my faith or religion? Am I violating my family's value system? Am I disrespecting my religious leader?

But we can also ask other questions. For example, Will I learn something new that will help replenish my belief or ideology? Will I make someone else's life better with my understanding? Looking for hope instead of fear pushes us to have an open mind while engaging with differences. It is often believed that anything unknown, remote, and alien is necessarily evil and ominous. This fear, however, is cultivated among people of a community through practices of punishment in order to discipline them and prevent them from venturing outside into uncharted ideological territories. This also implies that the act of inviting differences to a common table through shared conversations is risky and, many times, even dangerous. We might wonder, Why rock the boat? What if I am in a difficult situation because everyone else around me doesn't support my humanist views? Am I putting my children in a difficult or vulnerable position by encouraging humane practices? To mitigate these risks of holding difficult conversations with people, we list five strategies:

1 *Involve your family*

Families are our first solid connection with the community and its norms. Difficult conversations should begin with your family first. In India, many people have family WhatsApp groups, and more often than not, these are strong echo chambers wherein members feel free to openly express a prejudice or bias toward one or more communities, but progressive ideas are often attacked. If you have family members who use stereotypes or derogatory language toward other communities, initiate a conversation with them to understand why they harbor such animosity and hatred. Have they ever had any personal experience where they felt attacked by the other community? If yes, can they think of ways to unburden themselves with that baggage and move on? Can they be encouraged to meet more people from the other community, instead of generalizing based on a few experiences? Or you can just post a thought, experience, or meme that is the exact opposite, and drive a conversation through that. If your children post counterviews in a family group, that is a good moment to deepen your conversation with them. It helps to not radically attack or insult group members who think differently from you and put them on the defensive. Instead, tactfully, gently, and gradually drive the conversation to make your point. Just showing the other members that a counterpoint exists is a step forward. At the same time, be prepared to get your views challenged, and accept when someone else's argument has a valid point. Few issues are black and white in reality. Every group and community has problems and problematic people.

2 *Do not stereotype*

Stereotypes are over-generalized assumptions about a group or community which convert them into monoliths. Using stereotypes in conversations with others limits the scope of our conversations. Stereotypes can be extremely detrimental because they limit the scope of our conversations to things we assume we know about the other. For instance, one of the stereotypes and biases about Dalits in India is that they are unhygienic, lowly, or dirty because their families have been involved in sanitation jobs for years. This is extremely problematic because it limits our understanding of members of this community to a regressive, caste-based framework and, in a way, justifies their continued marginalization. Similarly, Black people in Western countries are stereotyped as violent and prone to crime, and this stereotype has a deep influence on their lives. Avoid using phrases and words that are intended to speak for the entire community in one tone and voice.

Examples of Statements with Stereotypes

- I have never met a Christian who questions the Bible.
- You are extremely non-aggressive for a Sikh.
- All terrorists are Muslims, right?
- Lower caste people are uncouth.
- Hindus are religious fanatics.
- Tribal communities are backward.
- Women bosses don't know their job. They better look after their kitchen.

3 Do not use humor to practice bias

We all know a friend, relative, or co-worker who uses humor as a way to practice and articulate their biases and prejudices. Cracking jokes that insult and humiliate a community is used to establish solidarity within social groups, as well as to draw the boundaries between them. This is the reason why such humor is enjoyed by the members of an in-group and not by the ones targeted—for instance, some of the anti-Muslim and anti-Hindu jokes circulating in our media. In our research with adolescents in India, we collected memes that were circulated in school WhatsApp groups. Some memes are disrespectful and make fun of the lifestyle choices, faith, and beliefs of a community. Taking a stand and voicing your concern over the use of humor as a way to normalize the practice of abuse is never easy, but it is very crucial. This is an important topic for family conversation, with children taking an active part.

4 Transcend your ideological boundaries

Start your conversations with an assumption that you know nothing about the other—and that could include your children and their friends or spouses! Ask sensitive questions, with the intention of understanding where the other person is coming from. When we do this, we learn many things that challenge our preconceived notions about the other, and make us uncomfortable. This sense of discomfort emerges from our fear of the unknown; uncertainties make us vulnerable and put us at a huge risk. Uncertainties, however, are also the steppingstones to transcending our ideological boundaries and exploring the world from a new position. Conversations must be built around the intention of knowing the other, and not on confirming our existing biases with more examples.

5 *Introspect*

The most challenging task in holding sensitive conversations to resolve differences is to identify when and how we practice insensitivity and bias in our own language and lives. How do people know when and if they are being prejudiced or biased? How do people withdraw or pull back from such situations? The first step toward being introspective is to trace the history of a thought—why do you think a community and its people are bad or deserve less respect? The second step is to evaluate if our reasons are based on stories of personal experience, or rely on the popular narratives we consume. Have I ever had any interpersonal relations with members of this community that made me dislike them? Or am I relying on "he said–she said–they all said," while making inferences about the other? The third step is to apologize and ask how you can improve and enrich the conversation. If someone from the other community feels hurt by your words and gestures, it is important to withdraw and ask for help in rethinking—What should I have avoided in articulating my opinion? How can I make this interaction more meaningful? Which terms, concepts, or descriptors would you prefer?

Conversations often take place in informal, more intimate spaces. The language of intimacy defines the core of such personal conversations and symbolizes a dropping of our defenses, making ourselves vulnerable. When people narrate their stories of lived discrimination in these conversations, they are, in some way, entrusting the listeners with the power to "judge." Though the aim of a conversation is never to sit on a moral high ground in judgment, every so often it happens that participants start forming an opinion about each other. As listeners, we must adopt a more generative style of meaning-making—an approach wherein, instead of making judgements, we visualize and interpret the narrative comprehensively, taking into consideration the history of interfaith relations, violence caused due to communal conflicts, and, most importantly, the cost of human lives involved.

Different Yet Equal

We have earlier looked at how some of the great leaders across the world have believed in and advocated for tolerance. We might think that it is not in the capacity of ordinary people, or the term "tolerance" may sound extremely philosophical and difficult to practice. Well, we never said it was a simple and easy process. But once we understand the term, and how powerful its practice can be for transforming our lives and our communities, it is not that difficult either. Again, tolerance does not mean we have to agree on everything. There will always be disagreement on various issues among people. Tolerance is the willingness to pay attention to other points of view.

It is, therefore, critical that we begin with a list of practices we can safely include in our routines, and leave out the others. We have a list of practices our readers can choose from to re-examine beliefs, recognize differences, and respect diversity. We suggest that each reader pick at least five practices they feel comfortable with, and includes these in their routines (see Table 4.2).

Table 4.2 Tolerance strategies

At home
Have an open environment for questions, debate, and discussion
Critically evaluate media, stories, humor, songs, and other cultural messages, involving your children in the process
Re-examine beliefs that have been passed down, and discard ideas which are rigid and problematic
Discard rituals which perpetuate discrimination
Accept that traditions and practices need to evolve and change over time
At school
Create a safe environment for questioning authorities and societal norms
Invite student discussions on relevant civic/political issues
Create spaces where different ideas and values can co-exist
Conduct critical thinking workshops
Create democratic and nonhierarchical classrooms
In our community
Increase representation of children in the organizing committees of religious and social institutions
Create spaces and experiences for intercommunity exchanges
Create opportunities to help older generations unlearn their biases
Create safe spaces for collaborative work
Demonstrate the merits of alternative understanding/perspectives

It is very difficult to include all these suggestions in our routines, but we can start by including a few, with the help of other family members. Once you have selected the five changes you wish to begin with, we provide a detailed analysis of how these suggestions can be translated into everyday practices of tolerance toward others.

Tolerance as Everyday Practice

In most societies, intergenerational mixing is diminishing. In conservative and traditional communities, children are often treated as dependents, and parents or teachers seldom grant them much space in important decision-making situations or discussions concerning family, community, politics, and so on. In others, even when families come together for social occasions, children and adults have segregated spaces—adults in the living room, children in the basement; adults at the dining table, children eating pizza while watching TV. In some societies, children still fear adults, while in others, they dismiss adults as an annoyance. Also, few adults apologize if they are wrong.

Critical Thinking as the First Step

In this section, we introduce an important term in the process of practicing tolerance—Critical Thinking—which is best practiced in an intergenerational setting. What is critical thinking? Simply put, it is a continuous process of updating our ideas and opinions, identifying faults and gaps in our understanding by opening ourselves up to fresh perspectives. As critical thinkers, we are constant learners, children and adults alike.

The hardest part isn't listing unfair practices; it's noticing them in the first place. A simple discipline helps: ask "Why?" of every rule that sorts, excludes, or shames, and then ask, "Who benefits, who pays, and what evidence supports this?" If a housing society discourages tenants from a particular community, demand the original rationale and the data—was the rule solving an actual problem, or policing identity? If a school's hair or headwear policy penalizes certain practices, trace its origins—was it written for uniformity, or to keep students safe around machinery, and does that justification hold for today's classrooms? Next, pair that with "Why not?" for plausible alternatives: Why not safety checks that don't single out culture?; Why not a gender-neutral dress code focused on function?; Why not opt-in photo consent, instead of public shaming for nonparticipation? "Why" exposes hidden assumptions and power; "Why not" opens a path to small pilots with guardrails—trial a change for a month, measure outcomes, and keep what works.

Relevance must also be tested against time. Many practices were born under different risks and resources: curfews tailored to poor lighting and weak transport, "English-only" rules meant to standardize instruction, blanket phone bans from an era before robust parental controls. Ask, "Even if this made sense then, does it make sense now?" Run a quick relevance check: Have conditions changed (lighting, transit, tech, laws)? Is the harm prevented still likely and proportionate to the costs imposed? Can the goal be met with narrower, fairer means (e.g., late-bus passes, instead of gendered curfews; clear-bag checks, instead of cultural dress restrictions; classroom phone lockers during lessons, rather than all-day confiscation)? Include voices most affected in the review, publish the reasons and the data, and set a sunset or revisit date so rules don't become fossils. Critical thinking, in practice, is this loop of inquiry, evidence, and iteration—asking "Why" to uncover bias, "Why not" to surface better options, and "Why now" to retire what history no longer justifies.

Practicing change: Let's understand how a change in our thinking is practiced in our use of language. We inherit our vocabulary from our elders, our cultural texts, and society. Language is, therefore, a conduit between us and our surroundings. If we wish to change our surroundings, to make them safe for people from diverse backgrounds to thrive, we can begin by using language that is inclusive and peaceful. Small changes in our language can make a huge

Table 4.3 Practicing nonauthoritative language

Instead of saying…	*Say…*
You do not understand this because you are too small.	How do you feel about this situation?
You are a child so act like one.	I know you feel strongly about this, but I would suggest you consider my advice.
You cannot question your elders.	We would appreciate it if you raised relevant questions and gave us time to address them.
You are not allowed.	Can we please sit down and think about the merits and demerits of this decision?
You have been a bad child, and you will be punished.	I believe we are not on the same page and are unhappy. I believe there is a lot of scope for improvement. Do you have any suggestions on what you can do to make up for this lapse at your end?

difference in our environments. When we use words that depict authority, aggression, and dominance, we create a hierarchy where some people feel uninvited or even intimidated.

In a conversation between parents and children, practicing language that is participatory and nonauthoritative may instill in our children a sense of responsibility towards the issues in question (see Table 4.3).

We can practice tolerance not only in the words we choose to interact with others, but also in our decisions related to the range of people and ideas we choose to engage with. Practicing tolerance can range from simple changes, such as modifying family norms in the house which favor male children over the girls, introducing a feminist retelling of fairy tales, changing the treatment given to household help, involving everyone in the decision-making process, listening attentively to other people's opinions and including them in the decision-making process, to complex practices, such as challenging the authority of archaic figures, ideas, and beliefs in your life.

Critical thinking skills are essential in every walk of our lives; they are the language through which we understand why and how our reality is limited, and once we know the rules determining the nature of our reality, we can modify them to introduce changes in our world. To understand this, let's look at the following conversation between a media educator and a parent in a city in Gujarat.

MEDIA EDUCATOR: The other day, Sheila was expressing some anxiety. I think she has some body issues and a very negative body image. Do you know something about that?

MOTHER: Ma'am, I have been trying to help her. Now the relatives are so eager to give advice and what we can do about it. We went to a wedding where my sister, her masi, advised her to join a gym. She is very fat, and how can she look good when she is fat. She does not want to diet. She eats all the meals.

MEDIA EDUCATOR: I am not sure, but is she eating unhealthy food?

MOTHER: No, no, ma'am. She just has 'ghar ka khana (home-cooked food),' but look at us. Everyone in our family has a weight issue. We are not a family of thin people. If she wants to look good, she should be very strict with herself.

MEDIA EDUCATOR: Do you think a better approach would be to make her feel comfortable about her own body first? Maybe later you can suggest she join a gym?

MOTHER: Ma'am, look at everyone around us. The girls especially! They are taking care of their bodies and looking good. They are thin and fair, and so groomed. This girl does nothing. She is fat, she isn't fair, and she doesn't care about her clothes. How can anyone be comfortable with the body she has. In fact, she should be uncomfortable. Only then will she change.

Given this scenario, critical thinking skills can help the mother understand three things:

1. Ideal beauty standards, i.e., who is good-looking, are created by the media, market, and popular culture. These beauty standards are very toxic, impossible to achieve, and promote a culture of consumerism.
2. A healthy body must be the goal. Beauty, as depicted through movies and commercials, is created by technological, medical, and other artificial interventions, and is not a healthy choice.
3. There is an alternative discourse on creating a healthy body and mind, and body positivity, which debunks the notions of flawless fair skin and the obsession with thin bodies.

Critical thinking is useful in exposing the fault lines in our world; it brings to the surface the rules and norms that make us and our societies patriarchal, divisive, violent, and hierarchical. Critical thinking helps us notice the hidden rules shaping family life—rules about work, gender, success, and "good parenting." It brings to the surface the norms that can make our homes and communities more unequal, judgmental, and stressful than they need to be.

Now let's give our rules and norms some more thought. Who created each of these rules and norms—some higher power or us humans? We tend to ascribe a label of "natural" to so many things that are just products of cultural practices. This leads to a recognition that the norms and rules are not natural or universal; they can and should be changed for the betterment of our communities. Our societies will evolve only when we can imagine things that seem impossible today. Critical thinking is a progressive strategy, a method to highlight the importance of unlearning some of our outdated values in order to create space for new ones to emerge.

In the following sections, we walk you through some interesting ideas to help with critical thinking that have been backed by research. These can be easily adapted to practice tolerance at home, in school, and in our communities.

Establishing Progressive Family Norms and Guidelines

We can use the "shared ground rules" approach, where each member of the family has the right to draft a few rules that will apply to everyone. Once all the members of the families have drafted a set of shared ground rules, the family can jointly discuss the feasibility of implementing these rules. Asking all the members of the family to create rules will help in enabling each member to prioritize their concerns and aspirations, represent their values and opinions, and learn to negotiate with the expectations of others.

This practice will then spread to our lives outside the home. Negotiating with other people's expectations, their desires and motivations, their goals and values is the cornerstone of a democratic social order. This process of accepting different voices and creating space for them to thrive alongside our personal beliefs creates a truly diverse society.

- In a family with a teen daughter and tween son, the daughter is required to keep her location available at all times, share her phone password, and hand over her device by 8 p.m., while her brother plays online games unsupervised past 10 p.m., with no history checks. The parents argue that it is out of concern for the daughter's safety, but she feels singled out and treated as "less trustworthy" because she's a girl. She proposes a family tech contract: identical screen curfews, the same rules for location sharing and password privacy, and weekly device-free hours that apply to everyone, not just her.
- The parents pay thousands for the son's baseball travel (tournaments, gear, hotel stays) and excuse him from chores on game weekends, but tell the daughter that robotics camp is "too intense" and ask her to babysit cousins instead. She feels her interests are undervalued and her time is less protected. She proposes an equal support policy: a shared activities budget split fairly, protected practice/competition time for both kids, and a rotating weekend chore schedule, so no one's commitments are automatically prioritized over the others.

It is a good strategy to pay attention to personal experiences and feelings of each member of the family, rather than dismiss them. They should be represented in the way family dynamics are organized.

Another strategy to create a climate of tolerance toward each other in the family is to initiate "Discussion nights," where family members come together and express their grievances with each other. Constructively expressing anger and frustration strengthens bonds of trust and feelings of compassion toward each other. This is an opportunity to introduce three progressive ideas in the family:

1 Vulnerability is empowering

Vulnerability is the virtue of accepting our weakness and asking for help. It begins when people seek out counseling, guidance, and mentoring when they find themselves incapable of handling difficult situations of lived discrimination in their lives. Many young students are bullied in their schools; boys and transgender students are beaten up, girls are slut-shamed, molested, or assaulted, they are body-shamed, and often pressured to follow their group. This can have a lasting influence on their psyche and lead to a loss of self-confidence. During these discussion nights, parents can begin expressing their vulnerability and seek their children's advice. Involving children in important decision-making processes will open a two-way door for the children to enter. Parents can invite children to share their insecurities and fears, and most importantly, enable them to deal with these challenges on their own. Most children are apprehensive about sharing their fears or problems because parents often assume the role of a "savior," swooping in, knocking at their school doors, and trying to rescue their children swiftly. Children argue that this is an offensive strategy because it makes them feel that they are incompetent to handle the situation on their own. Discussion nights are times when parents can assure their children that they will only be providing moral and emotional support, and will allow their children to make the final decision. Vulnerability, therefore, is also withdrawing from positions of power in our families and sharing authority with others. Parents find it difficult to give up their authority, to wait patiently while children learn their way in the world, and so they often resort to intervention strategies. The more we try to intervene and dictate terms to our children, the more they withdraw into their cocoons. If we wish to draw our children out of their rooms and into our lives, we must give them the space they need to think on their own, to act in ways they deem responsible, and to improve when they make mistakes.

2 Apology is powerful

Another value that parents must actively practice is the art of apologizing. In several cultures, parents seldom apologize; they rarely accept that they have been wrong, mistaken, or unreasonable. This is problematic for three reasons. First, children assume that apologizing is a sign of weakness, rather than a sign that the person is trying to unlearn wrong ideas, beliefs, and behaviors. Second, children start believing that power and authority render someone so powerful that they do not have to worry if their actions were right or wrong. When parents do not apologize, they are using their power to avoid facing the consequences of their actions. Children who observe such behavior can come to assume that power gives them immunity from facing the outcomes of their decisions and actions, which may encourage them to dictate terms when they occupy positions of privilege. Third, extending an apology implies an acceptance that learning is a lifelong process, and nobody will ever be too accomplished to ask for forgiveness and learn from their mistakes. When parents refuse to apologize, they convey a message to their children that accepting mistakes is a sign of weakness. Apologizing, and the process of learning from mistakes, are considered to be signs of powerlessness, rather than virtues in reflective thinking and personal growth.

3 Empathy is nourishing

The virtue of empathy involves two core characteristics. First, the habit of sharing emotions, where everyone in the family is encouraged to express how they feel. For instance, patriarchy in our families prevents sons and fathers from expressing emotions. Men are expected to toughen up, man up, and hide their feelings. This can lead to a lot of emotional blockage and frustration. Also, when men are discouraged from expressing emotions, they do not develop the skills required to deal with them. When they find themselves in emotionally turbulent situations, they either break down or remain unavailable. Oftentimes, parents and family members mock each other when someone expresses emotions of sadness, grief, and love. At other times, we push these discussions under the carpet with jokes or mockery. Children who watch this behavior may refuse to express their state of mind for fear of being ridiculed or ignored. Parents and adults must harness an empathetic concern, i.e., a sense of care and compassion, toward those who choose to unpack their emotions and reveal their vulnerable side to others. Attentive listening or listening to give advice or guidance can be very helpful in allowing children to unburden their problems and look for resolutions. Also, children will model their behavior based on their parents' practice of empathetic concern and will be able to use this emotional intelligence in navigating conflict situations in their communities, schools, and playgrounds. Empathetic concern is the ability to identify with the pain of others, regardless of their social identities, such as caste, class, religion, and gender. It is the ability to feel and extend care toward those who are suffering, stressed, oppressed, or vulnerable. Dinner tables, evening teatime, morning conversations on slow weekend mornings, television or movie sessions—all of these can be the most effective sites to introduce us and our children to progressive values and to implement these as a family. In the process, the family will have to collectively unlearn a lot of ideas and beliefs, as they meet the challenging requirement of upholding their moral obligation toward universal ideas of justice and equality.

Practicing Tolerance in Our Communities

Communities are our immediate circle of friends, neighbors, and relatives we spend our time with, especially during important occasions and events such as weddings, birthdays, anniversaries, sickness, funerals, and so on. The definition of community is fluid because we can have different communities based on our needs and identities. For instance, a Hindu family can be a member of a community based on their religious beliefs and identities, and the same family may belong to an elite club, depending on their economic status and position in society, and may also be members of a hiking club. On the other hand, a Dalit family may strongly identify with Dalit congregations and families in their neighborhood, as they question the Hindu caste system in India, and also participate in volunteer activities organized by religious groups, and the young boys of the family may be members of the local cricket team. Another case in point can be Muslim or Christian families who identify very strongly with their mosque or church congregations, an organization based on their regional identity, and are members of intellectual groups at universities. We become part of certain communities by default, given our social identities, but we can also choose to seek membership in several other communities that invite participation if our values and ideas align with their collective goals and ideology.

Our primary communities are those in which we gain membership based mostly on our birth, because of our religion, caste, class, and gender. Our primary communities are often extremely rigid and exclusive. Within these groups, members continue to reinforce the truth and belief systems dominant in their communities, and seldom engage with differences. It is also very easy to turn these communities into echo chambers, which can lead to people developing a myopic understanding of others. On the other hand, our secondary communities are those we want to gain membership of because we relate to their work and values, or because we enjoy doing certain activities together. These communities are flexible, more open to different ideas and people from different walks of life. In a way, secondary communities are more democratic and aim to create nonhierarchical structures of organization. Some examples include literary societies, film clubs, activist groups, online communities with participants from many countries, political outfits, volunteer organizations, social welfare communities, sports clubs, online gaming communities, and others. In India, we find several communities formed on the basis of members' love for saris, and globally, there are fan communities around a celebrity or a certain pop culture. In this section, we will focus mainly on understanding how primary communities can be made more liberal and inclusive. Toward the end of the chapter, however, we will list some secondary communities in which parents and children can participate in order to further their personal literary, political, professional, and other life goals. All the strategies and techniques suggested in this section are designed with the intention of nurturing intergroup relations and empathy in our plural societies.

Primary Communities: Diversity and Discrimination in Our Streets

Practicing tolerance in our communities begins with identifying how different tactics are used to keep certain groups out. For example, lower income people and women are not allowed to enter certain places or participate in some religious functions. Poor people are refused entry into multistory entertainment and shopping malls because their clothes and demeanor don't match the class requirements normalized by mall owners and goers. Gated communities are extremely exclusive everywhere. Conventionally attractive students, mostly girls, are allowed to present bouquets to the chief guest. These obvious practices of discrimination raise questions such as: Why do we do this? Do we have a valid reason to discriminate against people, or do we just do it unthinkingly because that is how it has always been? How do we change this? How do we feel more connected to those we see as different from us? Do we ever step into their shoes to feel how discrimination hurts?

Based on our work in different communities, we list a few strategies to increase representation and diversity in our communities:

1 *Let all voices be heard*

Many of our primary communities are controlled and organized by a generation of older people, especially men, who are often scared of change and constructive tension. For instance, in various religious congregations, older religious men take the responsibility of making rules and guidelines for everyone. They also assume the authority of counselling, sometimes coaxing, and sometimes scolding members into following community rules. Another case in point is the organizing committee in your apartment building or residential society that largely consists of older men who often refuse to invite participation or the opinions of others. Similarly, in women-dominated groups, older women normally take charge and assume leadership. As it is, in India we respect age and women are taught to keep silent when men speak, so this creates a hierarchy in our primary communities, and marginal voices, especially those of children, youth, and women, are rarely heard, especially if they try to challenge or suggest an option. Let's look at the following example:

> In a very affluent residential building in the city of Vadodara, a young female college student has invited some of her friends (girls and boys) to play table tennis in her apartment's common playroom. When the watchman saw this group of boys and girls playing together in the afternoon, he asked them to leave the table tennis room under the pretext that outsiders weren't allowed. This reason was untrue because the building guidelines didn't have this as a clause of compliance. On looking into this matter, it was revealed that the watchman was instructed by older men, who were a part of the apartment's council committee, to bar young girls from playing and spending time with boys without adult supervision. As is obvious, this was a case of moral policing, and the young female resident was extremely upset, as she felt that she was responsible enough to take care of herself, and so were her friends.

In this situation, it would be very effective to make the organizing and council committee more diverse and to include children, young members, and women in decision-making processes. Every day, we come across instances where our children suggest something new and we refuse to consider their suggestion seriously because we think that children and young adults are not sensible enough to contribute in meaningful ways. Similarly, in clubs and religious organizations, the wealthier a person (again, mostly a man) is, the more say he has. Why do we believe that if someone has more money, they will also always have the brightest ideas and the most appropriate suggestions?

This has to change. Our communities must be representative of different voices, opinions, and ideas. This can be done by creating opportunities to speak for those who are normally silent, either because they have no authority, they are in the minority, or they are considered outsiders or different. In a religious congregation, for instance, young children and adolescents must have the right to question the authority on the authenticity of religion and the concept of God. They should be included in discussions on how to change and update internal administration in mosques, encouraged to deliver public speeches that address the concerns of our contemporary plural societies, and to ideate projects for community service and outreach. Similarly, a young girl should be allowed to question unnecessary restrictions placed upon her during her menstrual cycle.

2 Make your communities accessible to outsiders

Various organizations that promote intergroup dialogue and engagement value practices that include granting equal representation and authority to everyone participating, avoiding the use of violence or aggression in words or actions, cultivating listening skills, and communicating with respect.

We can use these guidelines to make our communities accessible to outsiders. Encouraging community members to invite their friends, relatives, or colleagues from different socio-economic backgrounds to make acquaintances with the in-group members can be a liberating experience. For instance, let's consider a possible scenario in which we realize that some members in our communities belong to the LGBTQIA group, but are scared to discuss this with others. Every religious community will have conservative followers who refuse to accept that gender and sexuality are a spectrum. Many religious leaders are not willing to accept LGBTQIA people. People who rely only on a singular interpretation of their religion might find the idea unacceptable. In this case, some members of the community can suggest inviting people from LGBTQIA organizations to conduct workshops or informal sessions that encourage conversation on gender sensitivity, equality, and rights, without any pressure to immediately change views. Though such workshops and sessions will be uncomfortable for some people within the community, they will give them a new perspective to consider. Such workshops and sessions can also be very insightful for those members who identify as LGBTQIA, but are too scared to come out of the closet.

Another way to make these spaces accessible to everyone is the technique of sharing power. The authority of organizing and approving events in the community should be shared by different people. Positions of power must not be constant or static. Include everyone in the process of decision-making once in a while. This will ensure that more people with different values and ideas can express their concerns.

Finally, to make these spaces accessible to outsiders, try and build connections with different communities through collaborative activities. For instance, frequent different places of worship in small groups and learn about the different religious rituals performed there. Of course, we have to make sure we don't behave like careless tourists. Walking into a gurdwara will introduce people to the values of serving others and piety, time spent in a mosque will teach us the power of discipline in life and worship, and participating in an aarti at a temple can make us realize the effects of devotional music and meditation. Frequenting interfaith prayers can be a starting point toward introducing in-group members to ideas of co-existence and allowing for access to outsiders with compassion in their hearts. Similar exposure to people from other regions, countries, ages, interests, and political views goes a long way in initiating the practice of critical thinking.

3 Create opportunities to help older generation unlearn their biases

The older generation—our parents, grandparents, and community elders—finds it harder to let go of their biases and prejudices. As people age, they often develop a sense of loss—they feel that they are losing authority, power, and control over the new generation. This is completely natural and normal. In this phase, community elders cling very tightly to their old traditions and customs, even when doing so is against socio-economic development and positive change. Here, we don't claim that all the traditions and customs they subscribe to are regressive. There is much to learn from elders and there is much good in many traditions, but some have to change for our society to become more inclusive.

Such elders create a sense of fear among the community that the younger generation will lose their values and traditions if they are not coaxed into following the rules established by their ancestors, decades or generations ago. Such fear-mongering allows community elders to impose harsh punishments, and they are seldom held accountable for their actions.

As adults who support a more democratic environment, we can try a few tactics:

- Help create community spaces where everyone is allowed to express their opinions in a respectful manner. No one feels threatened or bullied because they hold different opinions. Elders should be willing to explain why they think certain traditions are beneficial, and be willing to concede if the younger generation do not find that to align with their current lifestyle. Our conversations show that when there is a merit to a practice, sooner or later, the younger generation sees it and adopts it.
- Question and challenge when members are punished for their personal choices, such as those related to whom to marry, have food with, or make friends with.
- Ensure a system where authorities change hands and no one is allowed to hold a power position for a long time. Encourage some like-minded members to advocate that everyone has the right to claim access to positions of power and resource distribution.

Unlearning, especially for the older generation, can be a challenging task. First, they do not have unrestricted access to information resources like the young generation does. Second, their exposure is limited to interactions within the community. They seldom go to places where they have no control over who accesses these spaces. They do not go to public places so often. Third, given how they were raised, they find it very difficult to apologize, and they also have a fear of losing authority and control. Not being needed anymore, being obsolete or irrelevant, is a fear that many older people face, especially when they have had a long stint in a position of authority, either at work or at home. Similarly, the younger generation should be open to giving a thought to those aspects of traditions that are worthy of emulation. Instead of blaming our elders for intellectual stagnation, a more effective approach can be to ensure they have access to information, resources, and perspectives beyond their comfort zone.

- Educate your parents about fake news when they send you a false message on WhatsApp or other social media.
- Respectfully call out the racism, colorism, anti-Muslim/Hindu/Semitic or other religious sentiments, hatred toward different caste groups, body-shaming or slut-shaming instances in group chats and family discussions.
- Encourage elders to participate in community services in their free time; put them in touch with organizations where they can meet people from different backgrounds.
- If our elders are mistreating domestic help or sanitary workers, call it out. Ask them to be more sensitive and kinder towards others.
- Spend some time with your elders, listening to their stories and also watching or reading narratives that challenge discriminatory social norms in our societies.

4 Create safe spaces for collaborative work

Community neighborhoods and spaces can be used for interesting collaborative work and projects. Collaboration over recreational, study, or work projects has been identified as a very effective way of nurturing relationships between different groups. Can we think of different projects where people from other communities can visit our neighborhoods and collaborate with people? Communities can seek collaboration over social work, such as providing food to the homeless in the neighborhoods, media consultation or help, educating children who live on the streets, painting the drab and dirty walls with attractive art, or putting on an impromptu campfire or an open mic night, and so on.

Personal experience with others can have both a liberating and a limiting effect. For instance, for Muslim youth who are already prejudiced against Jewish or Christian youth, or vice versa, one personal experience that reinforces their prejudice can push them further into the abyss of discrimination. It is easy to generalize and then use personal anecdotes to substantiate these generalizations.

On the other hand, when this experience with the other is positive, it can help both parties involved to shed their biases and perceive the other as friendly, or kind, or generous. If communities want to create positive collaborative spaces for intergroup engagements, they must ensure that:

- The organizing committee regulating these spaces has representation of young, old, men, women, and all different groups in the community.
- The committee weighs the risks involved in every project very closely.
- Every community member is aware of and encouraged to participate in these collaborative spaces, including in the decision-making process.
- The spaces and projects are conceptualized based on the "common interests" of people from different sections.
- Meetings, discussions, and other activities are held in neutral public spaces, so that everyone feels comfortable participating.
- Grievances related to bullying, isolating, ignoring, and suppressing are addressed with sensitivity and a sense of urgency.

Practicing tolerance at home, in schools, and in our communities is not a one-time commitment. Also, if all the groups don't participate in this process with equal dedication, no single community or individual can successfully build a tolerant society. Begin small, stay local, and constantly update. There are many ways in which we can contribute toward building a peaceful and tolerant society, and there is no one right way. The crucial point is that it has to be a collective endeavor.

5 Debunking Media Myths to Promote Self-Esteem

What do your children watch, read, listen to, and follow for fun?

Well, if you are thinking that by asking this question, we are encouraging you to snoop on your children's media use, that is not our intention at all! Yes, we want you to be aware of not only what kind of media content your children consume, but also what they produce. Not by snooping, though, but through conversations and genuine curiosity.

Reflective Exercise I

What is entertainment media? How would you describe entertainment media, such as popular songs, movies, television shows, games, and celebrities? Let's look at the following list of words and select the ones which apply to our definition of entertainment media.

Act	Creation	Artificial
Story	Glamorous	Fiction
Real	Constructed	Entertaining
Ethical	Morality	Lens
Depressing	Exaggerated	Technology

Now spend some time jotting down your definition of entertainment media. What can you draw from your everyday experiences? Which shows, movies, and songs does your family watch for entertainment? Why are these shows and movies entertaining? What do they do? How do your children entertain themselves using media? What is their media diet?

Entertainment media are media created and consumed for entertainment, leisure, and relaxation purposes. Though these media are created for the sole purpose of entertaining the audience, they form a large portion of our everyday media diets. Entertainment media can consist of a huge range of media formats

DOI: 10.4324/9781003590040-5

as well as media habits. To begin with, popular Bollywood and Hollywood movies, albums and songs, radio programs, television shows, and online games are all some of the very basic forms of media created for entertainment purposes. Of course, many more will emerge by the time Gen Alpha comes of age. At present, these media are channeled through television, movie theaters, radios, internet-based sources, and mobile phones. It is interesting to observe how the use of the internet and mobile phones has increased the scope of entertainment media, and new developments in tech will take it forward. We can now access international shows and movies on various online platforms. There are also Indian OTT platforms that offer more homegrown fare. The internet has, thus, changed the media habits of many of us, especially young people. Nowadays, besides watching shows and movies, and listening to songs, young people are spending considerable time gaming, and following, reading, watching, and engaging with celebrities and their online pages on Facebook, Instagram, X, and other social media platforms. The practice of scrolling, reading their stories, watching the vlogs (video blogs), posting, and commenting is all a part of the young generation's diet of entertainment and leisure media.

What's wrong with young people having fun, you might wonder! In such a dynamic environment, where the lines between the real and the fictional worlds are blurred, young people are increasingly influenced by what they see and watch in the media.

Why should we be bothered about the media diet of our children? Many young people mimic celebrities, social media influencers, and the culture promoted by the media. Also, a large number of media are produced to make money and therefore they don't like to challenge or displease people. Most popular media are produced with audience appeal in mind, and not to bring about social change. So, if they can create humor or sex appeal or drama by pandering to stereotypes, it is fine with them. These products, however, can leave a lasting impression on young people and affect their self-esteem.

An important area where media have strong influence on young people is body image.

Sanjana and her Struggles with Body Image

Sanjana is an 18 year-old college student. She has just started a relationship with her first boyfriend, Niraj. Sanjana and Niraj are both huge fans of Bollywood. Sanjana tries very hard to model her behavior, looks, and appearance after Bollywood actresses, as she knows that Niraj finds them attractive. She is in awe of their lifestyles, as portrayed through the social media pages of these actresses on Facebook and Instagram.

Sanjana uses lots of editing software to lighten her photos, to remove blemishes on her skin, and to look thinner in the pictures she posts of herself and, especially, with Niraj. In our conversations, she explained how she uses specific camera angles to make sure she looks thinner. Though Sanjana is not at all overweight, Niraj constantly compares her to the models and actresses. Sanjana follows a strict diet, and her mother complains that she often starves herself. Sanjana's college counselor has diagnosed her as suffering from negative body image. Sanjana does not feel confident in her body—she thinks she is fat, she does not have perfect skin, and has ugly features.

In our conversations, she often said she will get some cosmetic surgeries done when she grows up—she wants to enlarge her breasts, desires liposuction around her waist, and wants to get laser hair removal treatment done. She uses a lot of fairness creams, facemasks, and other products to lighten her skin tone and acquire perfect skin. She often refuses to go to social gatherings because she feels bloated and ugly. She has lost interest in academics, extracurricular activities, and sports. She thinks that playing sports will tan her skin and make her look bad. The worst of all, she is constantly insecure about Niraj leaving her if she does not fit the image of a beautiful woman the media have created for him.

Body image is our perception of our physical appearance, i.e., how we look, feel, and think about our bodies. Young people's body images strongly influence their self-esteem and, in turn, are greatly influenced by the media they consume. In our conversations with Sanjana, we asked her why she wants to lighten her skin tone. She said,

> Who would want to marry a dark girl in India? You think you cannot do anything about the skin tone, but that is wrong. All I need is some expertise and money. Look at all the actresses. Many of them were dark and like the girls-next-door when they entered the industry. Now, they are fair. Even all the popular international pop singers are slim and beautiful. That is because they invest time and money in their skin and bodies. I can get a lighter skin tone if I take care of my skin.

As she says this, she pulls out a tube of fairness cream from her purse and applies it all over her face.

A dermatologist from Ahmedabad discussed with us this obsession with fairness cream among young people in India:

> Young people watch these celebrities endorse this fairness cream all the time. These advertisements insist that if people are not fair, they cannot be successful, good-looking, or impressive. Then they see these actresses on their Instagram handles, or in movies and shows, without realizing that they photoshop the images to make sure that the "glam quotient" remains intact. So young people are being raised on a diet of glossed, photoshopped, and artificial beauty standards. The tags such as #summerbody, #bikinibody, and #bodygoals are often trending on Instagram, with millions of posts and followers. They develop unrealistic expectations of

> themselves—they want to wake up and look like the actresses look after seven layers of makeup and perfect camera lighting. They also have unrealistic expectations for their romantic partners. Girls, of course, have much more pressure to look a certain way than boys, but the media also makes boys insecure about their bodies.
>
> Not just the fair skin, cosmetic interventions now focus on breasts, nose, lips, eyes, vaginal tightening, and face contouring too. In recent years, my clinic has witnessed an increase in younger patients who want to change something about their bodies—they hate how they look naturally. This is troublesome for a simple reason that their ideas about "the perfect body" are unattainable, and to achieve these goals, they harm themselves. They will starve, apply a lot of harmful products and chemicals, go for unnecessary surgeries, such as breast enlargement or nose jobs, and so on. Parents do not know better, and in some cases even encourage their children to go for such measures, so young people rely on these harmful products.

The number of cosmetic surgeries taking place in India is growing exponentially. With plastic surgeons carrying out more than one million aesthetic treatments each year, India's market is expanding rapidly, and shows a strong upward trajectory. Young people participate in all these activities in some capacity; they are compelled to have diet plans and to lose weight in order to look appealing and to be accepted. This can result in several eating disorders and cause trauma to the mind and body.

Going one step further, when a certain skin color or physical appearance is given more than its due attention, qualified candidates suffer in job interviews, talented artists fail to get due recognition for their talents, and people even end up choosing the wrong life partner! Sad, isn't it? When people live with a sense of shame about their bodies, it influences every dimension of their lives—their education, jobs, interactions, friendships, and relationships. For instance, children who are bullied for their skin color or weight may refuse to participate in theater and stage activities, may confine themselves to their rooms, may refuse to socialize and attend gatherings, and may find it extremely difficult to make friends.

Parents also attach ideas of shame and dignity to the bodies of their children. If children use their bodies to engage in experiences deemed unethical by their parents, the adult narrative revolves around how their children have ashamed their families. Bodily experiences and experimentation should not be narrativized as "abominable," "dirty," "uncouth," or "shameful." In young girls and boys, for instance, masturbating is a very normal sexual activity, but many cultures stigmatize this. As a result, many boys and girls feel they have annihilated their bodies every time they masturbate. This shame could lead to issues concerning mental health and later sexual relationships.

The media play a huge role in creating an image of an ideal man or an ideal woman.

Media messages are then amplified by people in our surroundings—our parents, friends, families, teachers, and neighbors. Many young people, like Sanjana, who have a darker skin tone and are not slim are made to feel less beautiful, less attractive, and less impressive by their relatives, families, friends, and teachers. In our work as media educators, we have experienced many instances where children felt they were not cast in lead roles for school drama and stage activities because of how they look. In most of these cases, fair, tall, and slim students were cast as protagonists or lead dancers, even if other students ranked higher with regard to acting, dancing, and other skills. Similarly, in our families and neighborhoods, we have often seen elders tease young people if they are fat, or have acne or dark skin, and often extend unsolicited advice.

Low Self-Esteem Due to Toxic Beauty Standards

I was rejected in school and college for being dark skinned and I always remember buying men's fairness cream to treat this. Today, I am mature, and I have learnt to embrace my body, but those remarks still lower my self-confidence sometimes. I still do not feel confident wearing a white shirt because my mom used to say that white makes me look darker. She advised me to wear light tones which would not contrast with my skin color. Our parents and relatives also consume the same media, and they also start believing in the very same ideas. My classmates used to call me "Kaalia," "Kale," "Bhoot," and various other names. During the 12th grade, each student was supposed to have a date for the prom night and for that you must approach a girl. You will not believe this, but I thought to myself, "I will ask a girl who is the ugliest because I am ugly too, and if she is uglier than me probably no one else will ask her so she won't turn me down." Turns out, even she turned me down for a fairer guy. Now, this is so wrong. I was bullied because of my skin tone, and I used the same unrealistic beauty standards to judge my female classmates. These ideal beauty standards are very toxic. It is a vicious cycle.

Let's reflect: Which adjectives do you use to describe your children? Do you use any pet names for your children which mock their physical features, such as small eyes, long or short noses, chubby cheeks, plump bodies, heavy thighs, thin hair, or rounded bellies? Have you heard other parents, elders, relatives, siblings, and friends refer to young people as "shortie" (for short height), "uggs/ogre" (meaning ugly), "fatso/pudgy/whale/tubby/butterball" (if they have a heavy body type), "kali/kagadi/kolsa" (for dark skin tone), and other such slurs and forms of abuse? Have you heard your family members crack jokes about young people's body types, physical attributes, and looks? Have you advised your children to lose/gain some weight just to look attractive, or to use face masks and creams to reduce their tan and brighten the skin. Have you expected them to work out excessively?

If your answer to any of these questions is "Yes," it means our children and young people are being raised in an environment that promotes a negative body image and may cause detrimental effects to their emotions, psyche, and well-being. Let's spend some time on the following reflective exercise:

Reflective Exercise II

1. Sit down with a pen and paper.
2. List five instances when you have said something that would, intentionally or unintentionally, contribute to your children's negative self-image. Reflect on what role media have played in this.
3. Now ask your children to define and describe an image they would like to cultivate about themselves. Again, discuss whether any of this has been influenced by media and how.
4. List steps you can take in your everyday interactions to ensure that your children practice positive self-image. Look for alternative media products.
5. Create a chart to track your progress. Some indicators might be: How many affirmative terms and phrases have you used to boost your child's self-image? Which adjectives have you used to compliment, tease, or describe your children? What is your children's response to these words of positivity? Have you asked your children how they are feeling about their bodies and their selves?

This is not to say we should always praise our children, even when they do not deserve the praise. However, your criticism, even if valid, should be constructive. It should build the child's personality and confidence, and not break them.

In the following section, we explain how the linkages between media and people's life experiences create insecurities, doubts, and anxieties among children about their appearance their bodies. We also highlight how the media and society capitalize on people's insecurities to generate more revenue, customers, and brand desirability for products.

Media as the "Looking Glass Self"

According to the theory of the "looking glass self," individuals develop a sense of self based on how they believe others perceive them. People use social interaction as a "mirror" to understand their position, image, and worth in society. According to the sociologist Charles Cooley,[1] the self-concept is built in relation to others, in society and through conversations, rather than in solitude.

The Three Stages of the "Looking Glass Self" Theory

Stage 1
In social situations, individuals learn to imagine how they appear to others
Stage 2
Individuals imagine how other people judge their appearance based on various cues
Stage 3
Individuals develop a self-concept based on their understanding of other people's judgement about their appearance

In contemporary times, social media, for instance, is the most interesting example of a looking glass self. Every time we upload a photo, story, or post on our social media profiles, we invite others to respond, react, and judge our appearance and our looks. Sometimes, the number of likes or comments is a sign of societal approval. When many people like or comment on our stories and photos, it reflects how our friends and followers approve of how we look and present ourselves. The same social media can be used to bully others and reject their value or worth. Most young people experience instances of cyber-bullying and trolling through social media at least once in their lives. Similarly, they use their social media to create an image for themselves. They post about things they like to do, the products they possess, where they live, eat, and travel to. All of these posts and stories are ways of entering situations of social interactions and trying to understand whether our peers, relatives, or followers reinforce our self-concept.

Capitalizing on Young People's Insecurities

Companies manufacturing cosmetics, technologies, clothes and accessories, and various services tap in to the insecurities of young people to market their products and earn profits. Let's take the example of cameras with filters on our mobile phones. For many people, the most important criterion when choosing a phone is whether the camera has a "beauty mode." This beauty mode allows people to lighten their skin, remove freckles, make their skin look flawless, and sometimes to look thin in their photos. Young people are often insecure about their appearance, their looks, and their bodies. Marketers and companies exploit these insecurities, as they create a need for products that will help young people address their anxieties. In doing this, they reinforce these insecurities. Not only that, but unknowingly, young people start applying these unreasonable standards to others, and the vicious cycle of discrimination continues. Now brands also use virtual influences—influencers created completely using digital tools and having no physical presence. It is very easy to create perfect looks, bodies, and activities when there are no real-life constraints!

The expensive, high-end salons, gyms, clinics, and nutritionists who guarantee weight reduction of ten kilos in three weeks, clothes that make people look thinner, such as tummy tuckers, online services and apps for beauty tips and how to achieve flawless skin—companies, media, and the market anchor their messages on people's insecurities and create societal pressure among young people to align with the normalized beauty standards in their societies. Many luxury brands market their products as an aspirational value, i.e., people who can afford to own these products are seen as successful and have high social prestige. Let's look at the experiences shared by a young boy in Mumbai who was obsessed with the normalized beauty standards.

Of Brands and Money

I belong to a middle-class family. My parents work in a bank, and they work really hard to ensure that my sister and I have a good education. They got us into an international school in Vadodara. Most of my classmates belonged to affluent families, the super-rich families where parents spend very little time with their children, and to compensate for that they buy them very expensive branded products. That was the time *Student of the Year* was also released, and it was very popular among people my age. Girls would want to be like the characters in the film and buy all branded products. Girls who could not afford to buy these products or expensive clothes were bullied—they were called "verni" (i.e., vernacular) and all.

Being poor or even middle class was a stigma, and to avoid that you had to show that you were rich. I started pestering my parents for more money. I was always insecure about my looks—I am dark and short. I thought, nobody wants to be with dark and short guys. I started buying very expensive branded clothes to look more appealing. When my parents refused to buy me things, I stole them from their cupboards and all.

I was insecure and everyone around me made me believe that you can buy your way out of your insecurities. To be honest, that is not true. Your insecurities will only make you more vulnerable. To address your insecurities, you must work on them. My mother compelled me to attend school counseling sessions because she knew about my insecurities. I was always a very intelligent student, but all I cared about was how I looked and if I had enough money to "fit in" and to "flaunt." Counseling helped a lot. I realized that my worth was more than what society had put on me. I was good at studies, I was good at sports, and I loved reading. I always had something interesting to share and speak.

I also started reading a lot of inspiring books. *Wings of Fire: An Autobiography* by President Abdul Kalam is still my favorite.

Teenage years can be messy. Many parents complain that when their children enter their teenage years, they distance themselves from their parents. They do not share everything with them. This also makes it difficult for parents to understand what is going on in the lives of their children. In many cases of bullying at school, parents say that they had no idea their child was suffering or was being bullied. This is a phase when young people are developing a sense of independence, confidence, and exploration. They are curious about who they are, what they can achieve, and if they can make decisions on their own.

As parents, this is also a transition phase for us. How do we tread the boundary between granting them autonomy and guiding them? How can we set limits on the level of independence our children get to enjoy? And most importantly, how do we know what children are watching, listening to, talking, and experiencing without undue interference and snooping?

The Need for Peer Acceptance Online and Offline

This phase renders young people vulnerable to a lot of societal pressures, especially the expectations set by their peer groups. As a result, they succumb to the norm more easily and conform to societal expectations. To fit into their friend group, girls may start using a lot of makeup, even if they do not like it; they may start working out and dieting; and they may even go on dates with people they do not like or appreciate. Worse, they may buy into the myth, created by the media and reinforced by their communities, that boys don't fall for successful and ambitious girls, and this may prompt girls to underplay their ambition and accomplishments. Social media makes this situation worse; young people are constantly exposed to filtered images of influencers, celebrities, and their friends, and also look for validation on social media through likes and comments. It is difficult to encourage them to challenge stereotypes, discriminatory norms, and unfair practices because they want to be accepted, feel loved, and be included in their friend circles, school community, and neighborhoods. Many parents who have good disposable income unwittingly or willingly support their children's consumption sprees. If we want our children to stand up for what they believe is right, we will have to be parents and teachers who support them in this difficult task.

In our conversations with young boys from a school in Vadodara, one student said,

> It would be so much fun if we all could look the way we do on social media. We could do whatever we want with our faces—make the pimples and acne go away, get rid of the tan, and look super fair. I want to look like I look on my Instagram profile. I wish I were like these Hollywood and Bollywood stars!. They are ripped. They look perfect even at home. They #wakeuplike that.

We observe that social media, commercial movies and shows, and our society are pressuring young people to attach their worth solely to how close they fit the bill of an "ideal body type." As adults, we have failed at creating among our younger generation a sense of respect and love for different body types, a passion for fitness over "thinness" or "six packs," and self-confidence about their worth as more than just their bodies. Their intelligence matters, their skills matter, their hobbies matter, and their human qualities matter the most. Yet we are willing to ignore all these in favor of looks. The media have only fueled this anxiety. Our media fail to represent different body types in stories, songs, and events.

Anorexia and Bulimia: When Food Becomes an Enemy

The two most common forms of eating disorders among young people are bulimia and anorexia. In India, and globally, a sizeable number of teenagers suffer from one of these eating disorders. Bulimia nervosa is an eating disorder that is characterized by periods of binge eating, followed by either purging or exercising. Popular culture and our media have promoted ideas such as "thin is beautiful" and "thigh gaps are sexy." As a result, many young people now exercise more, while refusing to eat healthily. Anorexia nervosa is another eating disorder increasingly diagnosed among young people, where individuals refuse to eat food and often starve themselves to lose weight. These eating disorders can lead to several nutritional deficiencies and defects in young people. Adolescence is an age when individuals must have a healthy intake of calcium and protein-rich foods to build their bone mass. Bone health in adolescence is linked to bone health in later ages, and because of eating disorders, these girls are likely to have serious bone-related problems when they are older. If they follow strict diets and deprive themselves of nutrients, they may also be prone to detrimental hormonal changes and, in some cases, even heart damage and failure. When mother, cousins, aunts, and other adult women in their social circle reinforce the "looks are everything for a girl" myth, there is no escaping the beauty trap.

The media do not adequately highlight the effects of crash diets, harmful fairness creams, or other toxic products created and marketed to promote ideal beauty standards. Consuming media uncritically can ruin young people's relationship with food, their bodies, and their minds. How can we expect our children to accept their bodies when the only kinds of bodies they watch and see on their screens are photoshopped, thin/lean, and fair? How can we expect that our children will be self-confident when the media and society fail to acknowledge diversity in the way people look, dress, and present themselves? Should we hope that girls and boys will be confident in their skin when the media, celebrities, and influencers constantly animate links between

Fair → Attractive
Slim → Desirable
Curvy → Sexy
Six Pack Abs → Hot
Smooth Skin → Desirable

The question then is: How can we encourage our children to unpack the biases and insecurities built into these media products? How can we teach our children to love their bodies, to respect different skin tones, and to develop a positive attitude toward their bodies and their selves?

A different, equally pervasive myth shaping children today is the "filter-perfect life" that streams through short-video feeds and influencer posts. Beauty modes on phones, face-tuning apps, and AI "glow-up" filters present a single, poreless template as the default human face. The production mechanics are invisible: ring lights, softening filters, scripted "candid" reactions, and dozens of discarded takes. Children absorb the end result, not the scaffolding, and begin to treat comparison as self-assessment—my skin, my hair, my room, my grades, my friendships should look like this. What looks like harmless fun is a business model that rewards time-on-screen and emotional spikes; the more children doubt themselves, the more they scroll for solutions. The standard is global and portable—whether a child is in Lagos, London, or Lucknow, the same "before/after" template and the same soundtrack march across the screen.

This myth has social consequences beyond the mirror. "Aesthetic" friendships (beautiful people in beautiful places) and "hustle" posts (success without sleep or support) blend into a single narrative: worth equals appearance plus output. Children learn to curate, rather than relate. Classroom dynamics shift, as jokes target "real" faces or "uncool" rooms; sleep shrinks as late-night editing becomes normal; even kindness gets staged for likes.

What roles can adults play here? The fix is not to ban the phone, but to expose the production. Show side-by-side filter toggles and let children spot the changes; have them script a "perfect morning routine," then reshoot it honestly and compare feelings; teach them how to read sponsorship tags and the tiny "paid partnership" label; and normalize opt-outs—Filter-Free Fridays, camera defaults without "beauty," and family or classroom rules that require disclosure when a tool has altered an image ("Edited with X; skin smoothed; background replaced"). When children see the gears, the spell weakens.

A second myth travels through toy aisles and streaming menus: interests and jobs come in pink and blue. Superheroes smash, while princesses wait; boys "build" and girls "care." The pipeline continues in school plays and reading lists, where inventors, astronauts, and coders are male by default, and "helper" roles are feminized. Even nursery rhymes rehearse the script—What are little boys made of?— long before any child chooses a club. Global franchises amplify this split with merchandising and algorithms that push "more of the same." We have seen many schools displays where not a single woman is included among the tech leaders or well-known scientists! The result is not abstract: girls hesitate to opt into robotics or gaming servers that look male-only; boys self-censor interest in art, dance, or early-years caregiving because "that's not for us." Debunking starts with relabeling the shelves and rewriting the cast list. Rotate toys and tasks at home—every child builds, cooks, fixes, and cares. In the classroom, audit posters and examples, so that every unit includes women and men, nonbinary people, and professionals from multiple regions doing both technical and care work. Swap one show each week for content with girls who engineer and boys who nurture, and talk explicitly about why the swap matters. Children do not need a lecture on stereotypes, as much as they need repeated encounters that make a wider range of selves feel normal.

Parents and teachers can turn both myths into teachable moments. Ask three questions whenever media claims a "look" or a "lane": Who made this, and what are they selling? What work is hidden behind what I see? What else could be true here? Then practice alternatives on purpose. Document the "behind the scenes" of a school project and share it next to the polished result; invite a nurse who codes or a male kindergarten teacher to speak; run a "design your own avatar" day, where the only rule is choose for joy, not approval. The goal is not to shield children from media, but to equip them to read it, remix it, and resist its narrow scripts—so that what they watch expands their world, rather than shrinking it.

There are also steps we can follow in our families and communities to make sure that our children do not uncritically fall for media images, commercials, and stories. These include:

1. Using sensitive language: We cannot stress enough the role of language in shaping how we think and feel about ourselves. The first thing we can do as adults is to stop using stereotypes, skin-based slurs, and body-related forms of abuse in our families and societies. Emphasize that your child is beautiful, not despite their dark skin color but because of who they are as a whole person.
2. Increasing representation: Ensure that your children's media diet includes stories, shows, books, poems, and games, where different body types, skin color, hair, features, interests, and skills are represented with respect. Rely more on local narratives, i.e., stories which are contextualized in the child's context, with characters who represent the realities of families and people in your country and culture. Include books by writers from different cultures and countries, and not just from the US or UK.
3. Disassociating from "whiteness" as virtue: Make active efforts to disassociate your children from their obsession with white skin, sculpted bodies, and branded products. Introduce your children to young achievers who are dark, have different body types, are intelligent, sensitive, and beautiful. Equip them with information on how discrimination prevails in our societies, and how this discrimination limits them. Spend time with your children watching and critiquing popular media, especially commercials, and help them identify stereotypes and prejudices.
4. Discussing: Do not shy away from accepting and explaining body-based discrimination in our societies. Help your children understand how they emerged and how they continue to exist. Introducing them to other parallel movements against the "white ideal body type" around the world can help them gain a global perspective on the issue. Discussing the global movement "Black Lives Matter" can be a very effective way of unpacking for your children how race-based or skin color-based discrimination oppresses, limits, and controls us.

5 Intervening: Every time a family member, relative, or any other known person passes a negative remark about someone's body or skin color, intervene and explain why these remarks are derogatory, uncritical, and discriminatory. This may lead to uncomfortable situations, but if we do not learn to deal with discomfort a few times, we won't be able to change our cultures and our societies. At the same time, prepare your children to stand up for themselves and, in some cases, even ignore such comments and not let them affect their self-esteem. This is the most important role parents can play.

In the next section, we look at the different body types and discuss ways to cultivate a sense of appreciation for these differences.

Accepting Differences in Body Types

We are built with unique body types, features, and characteristics. The body positive movement promotes respect and appreciation for everyone and for every body type. On Instagram, there are more than 12.8 million posts with the hashtag #bodypositive. Body positivity argues that people should:

- have a positive body image and should be able to appreciate their bodies.
- be able to accept and appreciate differences in bodies and respect others.
- help build each other's confidence and acceptance of their bodies.
- critique and discard unrealistic body goals.

Body positivity helps people understand how their concept of self, bodies, and others is often shaped by social biases, other people's responses to our bodies and appearances, and the prevailing beauty standards amplified by media. Body positivity is a critical task of unpacking how popular media contribute to the relationship people have with their food, bodies, appearance, identity, and self-care. Understanding this relationship will help

Table 5.1 Accepting differences in body types

Negative Remark	*True Compliment*
You are very pretty for a fat girl.	You are beautiful.
You are dark, but who cares? You are so intelligent.	You are handsome and intelligent.
This dress makes you look thin.	You look wonderful in this dress.
This color suits you... You look fair.	I think this color looks very good on you. It makes your skin glow.
You lost weight. OMG! You look so nice now.	It seems like you have been taking good care of your body. You look fit and healthy.
You have gained weight! Now you won't look like a stick, and clothes will suit you.	You look very fit and healthy.

people to identify why and how they develop a negative self-image and body image. Most importantly, acknowledging why we think about our bodies and self in a negative light can encourage people to adopt new and more positive ways of engaging with their self and with others.

Human bodies are different, varied, and have flaws. The media-saturated world and, increasingly, AI-generated images make us believe that flaws are a sign of weakness, lack of discipline, or ugliness. Many studies have found that exposure to media messages portraying an "ideal physique" is linked to an increase in body image concerns and eating disorder symptoms. Body positivity helps us focus on all the wonderful things our bodies can do; everything we can experience because of our bodies. For instance, instead of being ashamed of their periods, young girls must develop a sense of appreciation for their bodies' capacity to create new life. Similarly, queer young people must be encouraged to embrace their uniqueness, their distinct sexual identity, and to channel their bodies to experience and navigate the world.

It changes our approach toward our bodies—from looking for faults and limitations, we start looking for strengths and qualities. Some of the steps toward body positivity include:

- Setting a good example for your children. Starving yourself, following crash diets, or continuously cribbing about your body is not helpful.
- Using affirmative language and appreciating your children and their bodies. Use phrases such as "You are so strong," "I like your skin," or "I like your hair. It's thick and curly."
- Normalizing flaws in your body. Tummy rolls, belly fat, stretch marks, or cellulite on other parts of the body are normal. Do not feel ashamed of it. If you have stretch marks from your pregnancy, it is a sign of courage and not a flaw.
- Following body positive influencers on social media, such as Instagram and Facebook.
- Talking. Ask your children if they are underconfident about their bodies, and why. Try to address their concerns. Help them acknowledge the talents that boost their confidence.
- Actively practicing complimenting and appreciating people with different body types in everyday conversations at home and in neighborhoods.
- Using fewer filters for your photos on the phone or at home.
- Watching movies or shows, or listening to songs that challenge the ideal body stereotype.
- Apologizing for every time you have called someone fat/thin/ugly, mocked people's appearances, clothes, or disabilities, and made your children feel that they are not beautiful enough.

No one should apologize for their bodies.

Healthy Mind and Self-Care

Can your body feel healthy and comfortable if your mind is not resting? We often ignore the "feeling" part in favor of what we can physically achieve and showcase. To be truly at peace with our bodies, to nourish and care for them, and to identify them as our homes, we must change the way we think about them.

We suggest adopting an inward rather than an outward approach when guiding our children in thinking about their bodies. An outward approach focuses on the role of your body in how it determines your role in society. This is a comparative approach where people constantly base their self-worth on other people's approval. The inward approach, on the other hand, encourages us to think about how our body helps us experience the world. Our bodies are sensory powerhouses: we see, hear, feel, taste, and navigate our environments through our bodies. Even when they aren't flawless, our bodies allow us to understand, explore, and learn. An inward approach draws force from feelings of gratitude and contentment. Let's look at the following activity of mindfulness.

Reflective Exercise III

Step 1: For a week, spend five minutes every day trying to use all your functioning senses. Smell your favorite scent, watch the sunrise or sunset, listen to the chirping of crickets, hold a hot glass of milk in your hands during winter, and splash cold water all over your face in summer.

Step 2: As you are doing this, think about the potential of your body. Appreciate the sensual possibilities it has to offer.

Step 3: On the last day of this exercise, define what beauty, happiness, and pleasure mean to you and how your body helped you enjoy these.

We can adhere to the following three principles to challenge the normalized "body standards" in our families, communities, and societies:

- Affirmation: Speak about yourself and others to build confidence. In times of self-doubt, reach out to people who will affirm your value and worth. Close relatives and friends who are sensitive and positive can be very helpful in overcoming phases of self-doubt and criticism.
- Intention: Make efforts every day to look at your body and self with a sense of gratitude, excitement, and contentment. Be aware of the many ways in which your body gives you pleasure and comfort.
- Action: Invest time in taking care of and appreciating your body. Relaxing and enjoying leisure activities are processes of rejuvenating your mind and body. Practice mindfulness and joy in the everyday things you do with your bodies. Do not abuse your bodies with negativity, overindulgence, constant comparison, or hate.

In the next section, we discuss a few exercises and steps to practice self-love in our everyday lives.

Self-Love

Remember the instructions we get from airplane safety procedures? Put on your own oxygen mask before helping anyone else. The same applies to body-positive thinking. We must learn to love and appreciate our bodies first, before helping our children and being kind to others. Loving and appreciating our bodies is a lifelong process. All of us experience uncertainty, doubt, and low self-esteem about our bodies once in a while. Maybe our skin has suddenly erupted with acne, or we have put on or lost some weight, or are experiencing hair loss. As we sat down writing this chapter, we realized how some of these insecurities are so deep-rooted that we have to constantly strive to unlearn them and to find new ways of loving ourselves and body.

So, how do we practice self-love?

Practicing Self-Love

Three elements are very important for practicing self-love, or any love for that matter:

Care, appreciation, and acceptance.

First, the element of "**care,**" which is manifest in the way we love and enhance the state of the people we love. Second is the element of "**appreciation,**" which can be witnessed in the ways we express our gratitude for what we love. And the third is the element of "**acceptance,**" which emphasizes that the things or people we love can never be perfect, and so we must find ways to deal with the limitations and focus on the redeeming qualities instead. We then decided to think about ways and everyday activities through which we can practice care, appreciation, and acceptance towards our bodies.

Care: Deliberate bodily abuse through indulgence is not body positivity. Many people misread the body positive movement as embracing unhealthy practices and lifestyles as well. If someone is thin because they are starving themselves, it should not be considered a positive attitude toward the body. Similarly, a person who continues to put on weight because they have unhealthy eating habits and a sedentary lifestyle is a problem. Being body positive is realizing that we have to make constant efforts to accept our bodies, as we strive to be healthier and more active. Eating clean, exercising, keeping a tab on our vitals, and making sure that our bodies are functioning normally are all a part of the routines of care toward our bodies. Care is practiced in ways meant to enhance and further the well-being and potential of our minds and bodies. If our lifestyle or dietary habits are putting our bodies and minds in the "inactive," "lethargic," and "sad" zones, we must re-examine our routines and change them accordingly. When we practice care in our routines, our children learn from observing our behavior. Some steps toward caring for our minds and bodies can include:

1 Right from a young age, make sure that children eat home-cooked, healthy food full of greens and fruits. Some parents encourage their children to eat from the "canteen" because they do not have enough time to prepare food at home. Doing this regularly leads to unhealthy eating and disrespect toward our bodies. One solution is to involve the entire family in food preparation. Children should be able to prepare simple lunches for themselves once they are pre-teens or teens. This is likely to contribute to raising their self-esteem too. Providing a healthy diet for the family should not be only the mother's responsibility. Also, parents can ration the intake of "junk/unhealthy" food for their children to once or twice a week. This will, however, require that parents follow the same regimen and eat at home.
2 Exercise with your family. Go for walks, practice yoga, or do other physical activities, such as playing a sport, dancing, or going for hikes. Plan active weekends and vacations, instead of spending those days in front of a screen. Encourage children to step away from the "screens" and explore the outdoors. Visits to parks, zoos, gyms, and yoga studios can be an interesting way of spending quality time together. Even occasional home cleaning could be scheduled for family time. Inculcate pride in doing home chores and keeping the surroundings tidy. With an increase in the spread of media and the internet, many children find themselves glued to their screens, playing video games or watching shows and cartoons. Parents also have the same habits of leisure and relaxation, which makes for an extremely sedentary lifestyle and can cause health issues. It is important to include 30 minutes of physical activity in our routines.
3 Ask your children about their mental health. In India, mental health is still considered to be a taboo subject. If people say they are suffering from mental health problems, they are either termed as psychos/mad/insane, dismissed as weak or emotional, or called dramatic. To overcome this stigma attached to talking about mental health, make sure you constantly ask your family members about their mental well-being. Also, in some cases of mental health crisis, family members or relatives are unable to help. In such situations, parents shouldn't fear getting help from counselors and mental health experts. Normalize the fact that the mental health of people sometimes deteriorates and weakens, just like their physical health. Normalize the fact that people can experience emotions and feelings they do not know how to deal with. Normalize the fact that seeking help, reaching out, and expressing vulnerability are very important for the well-being of both the individual and their families.

Appreciation: Expressing gratitude for our minds and bodies, appreciating how our minds and bodies help us achieve so many daily goals, and how they enable us to experience the world, is the starting step toward loving ourselves. Many health coaches and psychologists suggest a 40-day "mirror challenge." According to this challenge, people are encouraged to look at themselves in the mirror every day for 40 days and thank their minds and bodies for the things they were able to do during the day. We practiced this challenge with a few of our friends and family members. One of the participants said,

> I have acne on my face, and I am so conscious about it. The minute I step out of the house, I feel people are staring at my face but actually nobody even notices my acne until I bring it up myself, which I often do. When I did the mirror challenge for 40 days, I felt a little differently about my acne problem. I am still conscious, but now I have learnt how to distract myself and focus on other things my body can do. I am more confident while talking to people now; I can look them in the eyes, whereas earlier I used to try and cast my eyes away from them so that I wouldn't be watching them looking at my face.

Another exercise for appreciating our bodies involves practicing mindfulness. Being mindful of our body, the way it functions, and the pleasure and possibilities it grants us, helps develop a sense of gratitude for what we have. Let's look at the following one-minute exercises for practicing mindfulness toward our body:

One-Minute Well-Being Exercises

1. Stretch for ten seconds every hour: Every hour, take a ten-second break to stretch and feel your body. Stretching will reorient us toward our bodies and how we feel in them.
2. Stroke your hands: Close your eyes and feel your hands rubbing against each other.
3. Mindfully eat a raisin or any other treat: Sense the treat you are eating, how it smells, feels, tastes, its texture and consistency. Translate this practice to eating your food mindfully. Most importantly, enjoy your food.
4. Pray to your body: Twice every day, close your eyes and say this prayer: May I be healthy, may I be peaceful, may I love my body.
5. Mindful breathing: Every day, pause for a minute and count the amount of breaths you take.

Practicing appreciation helps unhook our self-worth from our appearance, and reorient us toward developing a holistic understanding of the role of mind and body in our lives. It is critical to delink our self-image from how we assume people perceive our bodies. Our bodies are meant to be more than just a "cover" and "appearance." Appreciating our bodies as a means through which we understand what it means to be alive; living is a blessing, and we must receive it as one.

Acceptance: Appreciating our bodies also includes being aware of how it is constituted: traits, features, characteristics, and limitations. Some bodies are thin and lean, while others are broad and strong. Some people have more melanin in their skin, while others don't. Appreciating how we are designed differently and how our bodies are unique is critical to identifying our limitations and weaknesses. We can always find a few good traits in our bodies. Many young girls, for instance, fall prey to the ideal body narrative and experience low self-esteem if their breasts are not big and visible. Many girls who have smaller breasts are called "flat tires," "planks," "blackboard," and other derogatory names in their schools and neighborhoods. On the flipside, girls who develop breasts earlier than their peers are also made to feel self-conscious and are called names. The first step toward challenging the "ideal body type" is to accept that different women have different kinds of breasts, and that healthy breasts come in varying shapes and sizes. Height, body type, skin color, hair, and features are all genetic endowments, and no amount of work can alter them much. Accepting our body, the way it is designed and structured, allows us to re-evaluate our expectations and bodily aspirations. Of course, we are free to experiment with style, accessories, and makeup if they help us feel more confident. The important thing is that these external props should not be harmful, painful, or draining on our pockets, and we should not accept them just to look acceptable in the eyes of others.

Caring for, appreciating, and accepting our minds and bodies will help us look at our lives in meaningful ways. It is important to remember that radical self-love helps us to embrace that #EveryBodyIsABeachBody, to make consistent efforts to maintain and further the well-being of our bodies and minds, and to seek help when needed.

In this chapter, we have only focused on how media and our social prejudices join hands in discriminating against people based on their skin color and body shape. Similar discrimination also happens when the media constantly portray certain communities, classes, religions, or castes stereotypically. Again, we have two weapons against this: produce and consume more sensitive media, and challenge such discrimination in our families, schools, and communities.

Gen Alpha is growing up in a digital world that is less a destination, and more an atmosphere: always on, algorithmically sorted, and increasingly shaped by AI. Their play, homework, friendships, and first experiments with identity all run through user-generated worlds, short video feeds, and chats. Real risks live there too. Bad actors have repeatedly tried to exploit popular platforms by slipping inappropriate experiences past moderation, luring kids to off-platform chats, or using gifts and "help" as grooming tactics. Add in newer threats like AI-fabricated images, voice clones, and bots that can impersonate peers, and it's clear that parental concern is not alarmism; it's a rational response to a highly commercial, fast-moving environment.

Conscious parenting is the antidote to both panic and passivity. It means being intentional and informed, co-learning the tools your child uses, and setting boundaries that teach judgment, rather than outsourcing it. It privileges presence over surveillance: sitting beside a child to understand a game's incentives, asking curious questions about a feed, agreeing on rules together, and then sticking to those rules consistently. Conscious parents prepare, rather than merely police, their children. They name values (dignity, consent, rest, honesty) upfront, translate them into visible routines, and promise help before judgment when something goes wrong, so a child will bring problems to them early, not hide them until late.

Note

1 Cooley, C. H. (1902). *Human Nature and the Social Order*. New York, NY: Scribner's.

6 Taming the Tech Monster

Childhood: Online and Offline

As parents and teachers, we have a love–hate relationship with technology these days. We are excited about the opportunities and efficiency it brings, hopeful about the bright future it might create for our children, suspicious about what it is stealing from us, and downright fearful about it snatching away our children from us. Well, love it or hate it, technology is here to stay; therefore, making friends with it is to our best advantage.

Identify all the statements which apply to your children and their routines

- Owns a personal mobile phone, laptop, or any other electronic device
- Is constantly in touch with friends
- Membership of online streaming channels
- Profiles on various social media
- WhatsApp on their phone
- Takes a lot of selfies and shares photos with others—publicly or privately
- Refuses to share their mobile phone or personal device(s) with other members of the family
- Loves spending time playing games online
- Has online friends i.e., people children meet and befriend online
- Uses their laptops and other devices for homework and education
- Refuses to leave their phone at home while going for outings
- Brings their device(s) to the dining table
- Thinks parents are too naive to understand why they are so attached to their phone and other devices

In our work, we have had a chance to speak with many parents of Gen Alpha. Their children's media and technology use, especially mobile phone use and screen time, came up as one of the biggest issues of concern and parent–child conflict. In Chapter One, we discussed how the ease and affinity with

DOI: 10.4324/9781003590040-6

technology define characteristics of Gen Alpha. As more and more functions in the world become tech-dependent and AI-driven, it is not even a wise decision to keep the kids away from technology. At the same time, overdependence on technology is associated with mental health and relationship issues, health problems, addiction, and diminished quality of life.

In our interactions with parents across the country, we have come across several instances where parents have expressed discomfort with their children being glued to their phones. Many parents complain that their children spend less time with them, do not enjoy face-to-face conversations with them or with guests anymore, and are easily distracted by their phones, laptops, and other devices. This fear of technology, especially mobile phones, taking over our lives, is particularly relevant in many upper- and middle-class urban families in India.

This fear related to children's use of technology, especially mobile phones and laptops, emerges from a sense of anxiety about the penetration and all-pervasive role of technologies, the internet, and electronic devices in our homes and families. There is no denying that these technological devices are changing our lives and societies, but this change is inevitable, and so we must learn how to embrace this new reality of the blurring boundaries between online and offline, the reel and the real.

Our children, who have access to the internet and technological devices, are now also online. Even from within the confines of their rooms and homes, they relate to ideas, people, and phenomena spanning across geographical boundaries and limits. There are both benefits and risks to children going online. Let's look at the following scenarios:

Scene A

Sohail is a 13 year-old boy who uses his laptop and mobile phone for educational purposes, as well as to connect with his friends and peers. He spends a lot of time online, even when he is doing his homework. His parents are worried that he will not be able to perform well academically if he continues being distracted by his phone and the constant online chatter.

Scene B

Rishika is a 14 year-old girl and her parents refuse to allow their daughter to use mobile phones at all. The family has a landline connection and Rishika's friends are expected to contact her on that number. Her parents have their personal mobile phones, but they do not use them in front of Rishika. Rishika often complains that she misses out on a lot of fun and interactions among her classmates on WhatsApp groups because she doesn't have a phone.

Scene C

Amyra is a 12 year-old girl who has unrestricted access to technological devices and the internet. She owns a personal phone, has a games console in her bedroom, and has profiles on Facebook, Snapchat, and Instagram. She has had some risky encounters with strangers online, but her parents believe in allowing their child to practice autonomy in how she wants to use the internet and her technological devices.

If we analyze these situations closely, we will realize that mobile phones and the internet are indispensable features of urban childhood in India. The question then is: How do we make sense of our anxieties, while encouraging our children to optimize the safe use of technology for personal growth and development? How can we embrace technology with the intention of expanding the learning, educational, and communication horizons of our children? How can we think about childhood and adolescence in relation to the undeniable presence of technology and the internet? In short, how do we increase their opportunities and minimize risks?

When children believe—and not quite unreasonably—that they know more than you about media and technology, you are no longer an authority that can dictate rules. This is the time to embrace engagement as an approach, rather than expecting obedience.

From Obedience to Engagement

How would you like a home where children do everything you want them to? They obediently follow your every instruction, are perfect in studies and high achievers in sports, and do all the hobbies and all the household chores with a smile. They respect your choices for them. They never argue, never question, and never criticize you. Awesome, right? Well, such a home is the worst place for a child to grow up and become a responsible and independent adult. Also, there is a high chance that the child's own happiness and self-esteem would be highly compromised. As Gen Alpha grows up, they will be facing a completely VUCA (Volatile, Uncertain, Chaotic, and Ambiguous) world, which technology and AI will be a huge part of. If you expect unquestioning obedience at a young age, they will find it hard to navigate the world as an independent and responsible adult.

Situation I

Neil is a teenage boy who fears his parents. His parents are extremely strict and expect their son to follow their instructions to the T. One of their rules includes prohibiting Neil from playing online games with his friends. They are afraid that Neil may fall prey to bad company, get addicted to gaming, get tangled up in scams, start consuming substances, and befriend girls. Valid fears, but Neil is so terrified of his parents that he never discusses anything about school and friends at home.

He wants to attend gaming nights with friends, so he often sneaks out at night without telling his parents. He comes home before dawn, and his parents do not know anything about it. The constant sneaking out and staying up till late is influencing his schoolwork and grades.

His parents think he is very obedient and focused. His parents do not know the reason for his poor academic performance. They are worried, but they have no idea what is causing him to lose interest and attention in his studies.

One night, as Neil sneaks out again, he rides with his friend on a motorbike and meets with an accident. He is so terrified of his parents that he decides not to tell them anything. His parents only find out when they get a call from the hospital. They are very upset at Neil, as they feel they have been betrayed.

Situation II

Rahil is a teenage boy who is top of his class. He has straight As and is often awarded "Best student of the year" awards and certificates. He shares a very open and easy relationship with his parents. His parents have set boundaries about technology and media in consultation with him, but they never punish Rahil. They ask him to reflect and think through his actions and to make up for his mistakes in some meaningful ways. Instead of calling for a timeout or grounding him, they encourage him to participate in healthy activities to make up for his bad behavior. He is sometimes required to spend some time cleaning his room/house, reflecting on the consequences of what he did and if he thinks it is wrong, helping his parents in their work. There are times when Rahil doesn't agree that his actions were wrong or unethical. In such situations, his parents listen to his arguments and reevaluate their interpretation. For instance, the school once sent a complaint to his parents that Rahil was bullying some of his classmates online. When his parents approached and reprimanded him, he explained that he was taking a stand for himself. He was, in fact, standing up against the bullies in his class who would mock and degrade him by calling him names like sissy, pussy, nerd disaster on his social media. When he threatened to fight them if they continued to bully him, they backed off but later complained to their teacher that Rahil was bullying them. When the parents heard his side of the story, they believed Rahil and apologized for assuming that it was his fault. They even encouraged him to go see the teacher and explain his point. Later, they discussed online bullying with Rahil and together they came up with a strategy to counter it.

Rahil has learnt to evaluate the outcomes of intended actions and is quick to assume responsibility when things go wrong. Even when he makes a huge mistake, he isn't afraid to own up to it because he knows his parents will help him make amends and remedy the situation.

What do we learn from these two situations? Situation I is an example of strict parenting, where adults treat children as unthinking, immature, and dependent individuals who need to be compelled to do the right things. In this kind of parenting, adults dictate terms to their children, and there's very little room for discussion, dialogue, or exchange. This style follows a top-down approach, and children find it difficult to express their grievances, doubts, or disappointment with their parents. Your parenting style can influence a great deal whether technology becomes a trusted ally or a troublesome monster in your family.

When children continuously receive instructions from their parents on what to do and not do, they find it difficult to develop their own sense of discretion on what is right and wrong. Strict parenting does not nourish the child; it scares them into submission, and then it becomes a lifelong habit to bow to power. Children's first encounter with power, therefore, is limited to instances where it is used to threaten and bully others. Also, such children would never use critical thinking when confronted with orders from someone in power.

Children should learn to associate power with a sense of responsibility and accountability for one's actions. Fear of adults and harsh punishments may compel children to control their behavior in order to please their parents, but such measures of discipline do not allow children the opportunity to understand when and why their behavior is unacceptable.

Strict parenting hurts the feelings of empathy, trust, and equality. That, of course, does not mean that there are no family guidelines about what is acceptable and what is not. Involving children in creating these guidelines, however, is the first step toward a more thoughtful parenting style, and it is a crucial step in shaping technology use in your family when technology, AI, and media are encroaching on the most private aspects of our lives.

Media Literacy and Education: A Helping Hand

The world over, leaders have found a simplistic and easy way to control children's social media and technology use—ban them. Many parents and teachers also support these bans, as it makes disciplining children much easier. Is this really a solution? There is a not-so-easy but helpful way of inculcating good and responsible media practices in children—Media and Information Literacy (MIL). As parents of Generation Alpha, we are raising children in an environment where digital devices, online platforms, and AI-powered technologies are not just tools, but integral parts of their daily lives. Unlike previous generations, our children encounter media from their earliest years—learning, socializing, and even playing in spaces shaped by algorithms and constant connectivity. This reality makes it impossible to shield them completely through bans or restrictions; instead, we need to provide them with the skills to navigate these spaces responsibly. MIL including AI literacy offers precisely this foundation, ensuring that our children can critically evaluate what they see, hear, and share online.

At its heart, MIL is about more than understanding how to use technology; it is about developing a deeper awareness of how media work, who controls them, and what purposes they serve. For our children, this also means recognizing when information is trustworthy and when it might be manipulative, learning how algorithms shape what content appears on their screens, and understanding the implications of sharing personal data. By incorporating elements like digital literacy, algorithmic literacy, and AI literacy, MIL gives young people the tools to see through the surface of technology and become active and informed participants, rather than passive consumers. As parents, this is critical: we want our children not only to be safe, but also empowered to make decisions that reflect their values and protect their well-being.

The role of MIL in raising Gen Alpha is ultimately about preparing them for a future in which technology will be even more pervasive and powerful. Teaching our children these skills helps them resist harmful content, avoid the traps of misinformation, and use digital platforms as spaces of creativity, learning, and connection. More importantly, it fosters resilience, ensuring they do not feel powerless in the face of overwhelming information flows or emerging technologies like generative AI. As parents, embracing Media and Information Literacy is our way of equipping our children with lifelong skills that not only protect them, but also enable them to thrive, advocate for themselves, and contribute thoughtfully to the digital societies they are inheriting.

The role of MIL extends beyond personal empowerment, to shaping democratic participation and social resilience. By teaching children and adults how media ecosystems operate—how algorithms curate feeds, how data is monetized, and how synthetic media, like deepfakes, blur truth and fabrication—MIL prepares them to engage thoughtfully with technology, rather than fear it. Unlike bans, which create avoidance and disengagement, MIL emphasizes agency, equipping learners with tools to protect themselves, advocate for accountability, and harness digital media for self-expression and collective action. In this way, MIL is not merely a protective measure, but a foundational skill for living and thriving in the information society.

In India, very few schools have a media literacy or education curricula designed to equip young people with the critical skills required to understand that media images, stories, and posts can be cleverly constructed, are artificial, and are not reality, even for those who create them. Media, information, and AI literacy help children and adults alike in evaluating, producing, and using these tools critically and to their benefit. Such literacy is a crucial life skill for Gen Alpha and their parents alike because, while many things about childhood have stayed constant over the years, many more have changed drastically. And as we discussed earlier, technology, the internet, and AI are huge driving forces in transforming Gen Alpha's childhood experience compared to previous generations.

The New Childhood

Childhood is now a phase when children are surrounded by technologies in their homes, schools, and communities, and by that logic, they are always connected to people, ideas, and events beyond their immediate reach. Parental control becomes challenging. Constant exposure to unrestricted information and connections is influencing childhood experiences for our children in three significant ways:

1 Children are spending more time developing and nurturing relationships and connections virtually or with their technologies, and this can have some influence on their ability to hold and engage in face-to-face communication and hold conversations in their lives. Many youngsters prefer to interact with a chatbot and seek advice from it, rather than the humans in their lives. Face-to-face conversations during childhood are critical for children to develop empathy and sensitivity toward their families, communities, and societies. If a balance is not maintained, face-to-face conversations will be eclipsed by virtual connections, and children will find it difficult to learn and interpret social cues, emotions, and gestures integral to the conversational nature of human societies.

   Can you imagine what would happen if a child were constantly interacting with technological/voice-based assistants? They would assume that a normal pattern of interaction is that they ask and the other answers, they command and the other obeys. Such children would find it difficult to deal with human interaction, where they would be questioned, challenged, or ignored; where the response is not always immediate and they have to wait for a response; where they cannot fast forward the parts they find boring! Online interactions foster different kinds of communication skills, but spending considerably long amounts of time with technological devices and away from real, offline social interactions can not only hinder the development of relational skills among children, but also encourage them to make negative progress.
2 Childhood is no longer limited to what can be accessed or experienced physically. This includes the experiences through augmented and virtual realities (AR and VR), the overflow of information, and access to multiple sources of entertainment and education available at the click of the button. Indiscriminatory use of this can overwhelm children and their parents, but judicious use can allow them to expand their horizons of knowing and communication. The risks in online encounters are real, but so are the opportunities to grow and become a better human being. For instance, the time children spend on the internet can be used to introduce them to different realities in the world, to connect them with people from different cultures and regions, albeit in a safe way, or it may lead them to create echo chambers and replicate their offline networks in their online worlds.
3 Virtual connections and digital networks can redefine offline realities for many children, as they may grant them access to skills, opportunities, mentors, and learning experiences that otherwise may have been inaccessible to them. This can produce significant positive changes in their lives. For instance, many organizations organize and hold online contests, conferences, and workshops, inviting children from across the country and the

globe to participate in meaningful experiences. Also, the internet enables a low capital-intensive environment where children can learn to use digital tools and techniques to create, play with, and implement novel ideas related to issues of their interests. For instance, many young people in India appreciate Japanese anime, K-pop, and BTS, and are actively involved in online social activism and justice. We also see many examples of youngsters whose proficiency in AI has set them on an early and successful entrepreneurial journey.

Technologies, especially smartphones and GenAI, which foster connection and exchanges anytime, anywhere, have become an inevitable part of children's everyday lives. In the following section, we draw special attention to the role of the internet and digital networks in the everyday lives of children in India.

The Internet, AI, and Everyday Life

The internet defines all aspects of the lives of our children, more so after the pandemic, and AI is already a force to be reckoned with. In March 2020, when the entire world was dealing with the COVID-19 pandemic, most countries announced a lockdown, and children were confined to their homes. Every aspect of our offline lives went online—schools, work, shopping, entertainment, family gatherings, game nights, and conversations. Though the effects of the pandemic have been brought under control and the world is opening up, the COVID-19 lockdown has shaped a generation of children, for whom the internet will be the most significant mediating platform for connection and communication across regions and ideologies.

Have we given enough attention to how our children will be raised in a world that is increasingly defined by the internet, virtual communities, digital networks, and AI? Can we create home environments conducive to such a technologically developed possibility? Or are we scared that such a world, replete with unimaginable possibilities, will destroy human societies and relations? These anxieties have exponentially increased with reference to AI and how it will affect our children's future.

The proliferation of the internet and digital networks has rendered the entire world accessible to children with smartphones and internet connections. Let's consider the flow of media products from different countries of the world to India through various online streaming platforms. Here, the circulation of media products also entails exposure to different cultures, societies, and realities represented through those narratives. For instance, many young children in India are familiar with Japanese culture because they regularly consume anime. These children are often a part of online anime fan communities, consisting of members from across the world, belonging to different regions, religions, and societies, and speaking different languages. Children develop meaningful relationships through such interactions, and their ideas about themselves—who they are, where they belong, and what their priorities in life are—are informed by these online interactions and friendships. Yes, if we are controlling parents and think that our culture and religion are the best with no flaws and that exposing children to different ideas would undermine our control, we will look at this reality with fear and suspicion. Unfortunately, there is no way to control this reality, but there are ways to face it wisely and meaningfully. There are also fun and meaningful ways to develop interest in our own cultures.

In the following section, we will explore how children's engagement with the internet influences their identity and understanding of the world.

In India, many parents are at a loss when their tech-savvy children throw technological and internet-based jargon at them. For instance, let's look at the experience of a mother with two teenage children who are constantly glued to their phones and laptops.

Keeping Up with the Kids

As soon as my children got their personal phones and study laptops, they started talking in a totally different language. When I say language, I also mean that their lifestyle changed, and I could not connect with them anymore. They stopped watching TV with us (parents) in the living room. They spent more time in their bedrooms, talking to their friends on video calls.

I remember, I was calling out for my daughter to come join us for dinner one day when she texted me from her room which is literally ten steps away from the dining area and told me that she is going to bed. She finished her text with "ttyl."

I lost my cool. I had spent so much effort cooking that dinner for them and they could not step out of their rooms and away from their phones to tell me that they were not hungry. In the spur of the moment, I got very angry with her but on further reflection, I realized two things. Mobile phones are changing our understanding about privacy and intimacy. They are also changing the way we talk—the words, sentences, emotions, gestures we use through our phones. If I must keep up with this changing generation, I cannot shy away from technology. I may not be a "pro" at it like these kids who have grown up with technology are, but I can learn to use these devices to my advantage.

When parents refuse to remain updated about new technologies, they create a "generational distance" between themselves and their tech-savvy children. This distance generally manifests in children deciding to override parental authority in issues related to technology use, such as the time they should spend with their gadgets, things they should do online, people they should befriend, the appropriate and ethical use of AI, and so on. As parents and educators, we must keep abreast of technological advancements, learn how to use the internet and social media in meaningful ways, know where AI is heading to help children become more sensitive and socially aware individuals, and guide them away from dangerous terrains, such as plagiarism, cyberbullying, identity theft, fake information, and online hate. It is not necessary to learn every new app or AI tool, or to be an expert gamer. Of course, as adults, we have other priorities and interests. It helps, however, to know the basics, so that we can engage in conversations with our children and don't always see their internet use with suspicion and resentment. In what follows, we describe ways in which parents can become tech-savvy and help their children conquer the realm of the internet and social media platforms.

Becoming a Tech-Savvy Parent

From the Journal of a 40-Year-Old Mother in Bangalore

My daughter is nine years old, part of the so-called Gen Alpha, and she is growing up in a world where TikTok reels, AI chatbots, and online gaming are as normal for her, as textbooks once were for me. I often find her clicking through videos or apps so quickly that I can hardly keep up, and while she is sharp, there are moments when I realize she doesn't always know which links to trust or what information is safe to share. Sometimes she turns to her cousins for help, but like all kids, if they're not on good terms that day, she's left figuring things out on her own.

During the 2023 floods in Bangalore, when schools shut down for weeks, her classes were moved entirely online. I thought she was diligently attending lessons, but I later discovered she had been using a second browser window to watch videos while her teacher spoke on Zoom. She assumed I wouldn't notice because, in her words, "Mom doesn't really get how these things work." I felt a pang of guilt—I had been working from home too, juggling office meetings on Teams and struggling to keep up with new software myself. After a frustrating day, I decided to sit down and learn, and also to talk to my daughter about her behavior. With a few YouTube tutorials, I figured out how to install parental controls, block distracting sites, and even set up time limits on her tablet.

That experience taught me something important: if we don't learn how to navigate these technologies ourselves, our children will stay one step ahead, leaving us unable to guide or protect them. More than rules or bans, what they need is for us to walk alongside them—to understand the digital spaces they live in, to build trust, and to teach them how to stay safe and thoughtful in a world where the internet is not just a tool, but a way of life.

The Stranger Danger

Now there is a serious parenting dilemma. Should we allow our children to connect with communities and people we do not know in the offline world, or should we insist they use the internet and social media to connect only with people we are familiar with? If we choose the first option, there is a good possibility that we and our children will use the internet and social media to create a new and safe public space, where people can think through ideas, concepts, and strategies to further their aspirations. At the same time, the internet is full of harmful people too—pedophiles, sexual abusers, scamsters, extremists, and bullies—and there is a good chance we will encounter some of these when we are online. If we use the internet only to remain in touch with people we already know, however, we are not making the best use of its potential.

Before we plunge into this discussion, let's examine the role of the internet and social media platforms in initiating and sustaining discussions, deliberations, and activism, and in creating supportive communities.

The internet and social media are now recognized as virtual public spaces where large-scale networks can be forged and young people can learn critical conversational skills. These are great places to develop what we call a "public voice." Children use their social media profiles to create an identity they want to project for themselves. They use their profiles and networks to communicate who they are, what they believe in, and who they wish to connect with. The simple act of posting, responding to other people's posts, sharing information, discussing, and creating new content to argue and present their opinions, ideas, or stories can enable them to practice autonomy. Virtual communities also provide nurturing spaces for those children who do not find adequate support in their local communities. For instance, a gay child in India may find it difficult to find support groups and networks within their own immediate local communities. In such cases, virtual support groups, friendships, and mentorship over social media platforms and the internet can prove to be very effective in helping the child make sense of their feelings, emotions, mental conflicts, and other issues. Similarly, many young people resort to the internet to read, study, and understand practices of "safe sex" because their family members do not feel comfortable talking about sexual health with them.

Let's Look at some Other Similar Cases

1 Shreenita is a 16-year-old girl who lives in Mumbai. She loves arts and crafts and wants to dedicate more time to learning how to paint. Both her parents have a 9-to-5 job schedule and do not have the time or energy to take her to an arts and crafts class after school. Shreenita decided to join a Facebook group where she attends free live sessions with arts and crafts instructors who teach young people different skills regularly. She has also made friends with other members from the US, Spain, and Singapore. They have created a five-member group online, and they share their arts and crafts items with each other regularly.

2 Rakesh, a 15-year-old boy from Mumbai, is a member of an international WhatsApp cooking group where the group admin—a famous chef—posts recipes of different cuisines and encourages the members

from different countries to experiment with them and to send their feedback. He has learned how to bake, grill, and make gourmet dishes from this online group, all for free.

3 Miss Bernie is a high school teacher in Ahmedabad and she has created a WhatsApp group where she posts sample question papers, quiz exams, and interesting resources to help her students. Using WhatsApp allows Miss Bernie to interact with her students and discuss educational topics, even after class hours.

In all these cases, children, teachers, and parents use the internet to overcome geographical or other practical barriers to learning, communicating, and networking. Such communities are usually safe, some of them are also moderated, and one should also take extra care in ensuring that our children learn safe use of the internet.

How to Be Safe in an Interconnected World

Before we plunge into devising ways to protect our children from the perils of internet use and social media, let's understand these possible threats in detail. Many children with access to the internet and social media experience some form of cyberbullying, cyberthreats, or breach of privacy issues. In some other cases, these children are themselves online offenders—harassing, bullying, and threatening others. The technological possibilities afforded by social media—especially anonymity and the resulting deniability/distance—may embolden many young people and adults to undertake offensive and criminal activities online.

There are five main forms of online abuse and exploitation that we need to be aware of:

1 Cyberbullying: This includes emotional harassment, social exclusion, defamation, social exposure or revelation of private details, and intimidation.
2 Online sexual abuse: The circulation of sexually explicit messages about someone, leaking their personal photos or videos, making rape threats, and revenge porn, using AI-generated images and cheap fakes to malign their reputation.
3 Cyber extremism: Ideological indoctrination, threats of violence, and encouraging children to become violent.
4 Online commercial fraud: Identity theft, hacking, phishing, financial fraud. Here, phishing refers to the fraudulent practice of sending emails purporting to be from reputable companies in order to persuade individuals to reveal personal information. Similarly, catfishing is the practice of creating a fake online persona to communicate with others on social media.
5 Grooming: Preparing a child and their environment for sexual abuse and exploitation.

Gen Alpha will also encounter these threats more than once in their digital childhoods. Ordinary tools of media production and distribution in the hands of ordinary users can also become high stakes. Sexting is a prime example of this. Among tweens and teens, it spans a spectrum—from curious, consensual exchange, to pressured, coerced, or criminal behavior—and the lines blur fast when screenshots travel, group chats pile on, or an adult masquerades as a peer. These media require special conversations.

Families and schools should separate three issues in these conversations: consent (no image without an enthusiastic "yes," and "no" is final); control (once sent, you may lose it; that risk should be named openly); and coercion (pressure, threats, bribes, or secrecy demands make it abuse, not romance). Practical habits help: turn off auto-save to cloud albums you share with family accounts; teach "exit scripts" kids can use ("I'm not sending pictures—let's talk about something else," "I don't keep secrets that make me uncomfortable"); normalize asking for help without blame; and treat forwarding, mocking, or storing someone else's image as a serious breach of trust, with consequences at home and at school.

GenAI raises the stakes by lowering the cost of harm. Face-swap "nudes," AI-cloned voices, and AI-written flirty chats can be used to harass, impersonate, or extort—even when the target never took or sent an image. This is sexual- and gender-based abuse dressed up as "tech." Kids and caregivers need to learn about the new red flags: sudden requests to move to a private app, demands for money or more images under threat of exposure, voice notes that sound right but come from new numbers, and profiles that recycle stock photos.

Adults need to devise a clear playbook to avoid harm in such cases:

- Stop engaging.
- Save evidence.
- Block and report on-platform.
- Tell a trusted adult the same day.

Schools need to adopt disclosure norms ("If AI helped create media, say so"), include non-consensual deepfakes in anti-bullying policies, and pre-identify escalation paths—to the platform, to school leadership, to law enforcement where threat or extortion is present. Media and Information Literacy also means that families learn to lock down discoverability and DMs, regularly review friend lists, and agree in advance that if something goes wrong, the priority is safety and containment, not punishment.

Gender dynamics still shape who is targeted and how. Girls, LGBTQIA youth, and gender-nonconforming students are disproportionately harassed or threatened with image-based abuse; boys are more often shamed out of seeking help. Meet these patterns head-on. Retire victim-blaming language. Replace "Why did you…?" with "Thank you for telling me—let's fix this." Make space for boys to report pressure without jokes about masculinity. Teach everyone to be an active bystander: don't forward, don't like, don't comment; do save evidence, do report, do check on the person being targeted. Schools can run brief, repeated advisory drills: identify a fake, write a refusal text, practice a report, and role-play supporting a friend.

We must include a note here on enormous platforms for user-generated games. Most play is harmless; however, bad actors have repeatedly tried to exploit the scale—through inappropriate "condo" experiences that slip past moderation, invites to off-platform chats, role-plays that edge into sexualized content, and grooming behaviors masked as "help" or "gifts." Treat such platforms like public spaces with kids' areas, rather than a sealed nursery. Here are some measures you can take to ensure kids' safety on such platforms:

- Use account restrictions and age verification
- Disable or limit chat and who can message, friend, or join games
- Keep play in shared family spaces
- Set spend limits and alerts
- Steer children to known developers or private servers with real-life friends
- Review the "recently played" list and friend list together monthly
- Teach the rule "Never move to another app or accept gifts from strangers"
- Practice the trio kids need to recall under stress: leave, block, report—then tell an adult

The goal isn't to ban every platform; it's to raise platform-literate kids who can spot grooming patterns, exit early, and trust that adults will help without shame. Instead of panicking and banning internet use for children, it is always better to educate them about ways to protect themselves against dangers on social media. We know that crossing the road involves the risk of getting hit by a vehicle, but we don't stop our children from crossing the road ever, do we? We hold their hands in the beginning, teach them how to do it safely, and make them aware of the rules. It is the same with the internet.

We have mentioned several specific guidelines earlier in this chapter. As an overarching practice, we suggest a three-pronged approach to enable our children to counter social media threats.

a Internet and AI discipline.
b Transparency.
c Digital literacy.

Let's look at each in detail.

Internet and AI Discipline

It is impossible to keep our children away from the internet, and especially social media. With all the kinds of possibilities that generative AI now offers, leisure time is increasingly being spent on devices. When children have access to technologies, the internet, and social media, they sometimes refuse to accept the authority and experience of their elders—teachers and parents—in learning how to navigate these gadgets and networks. They also think that they know more than us! The first step toward protecting children from social media threats is to create a routine of discipline. It is advised that parents be aware of their children's internet-based social media activities and practices. Many educators suggest using shared devices for education and entertainment until the child reaches 16 years of age or more. Instead of granting your child a personal laptop, parents can consider installing a desktop in a shared space—the study room—which can be accessed by all members of the family. The second strategy can involve deciding together on the number of hours children are supposed to spend on their gadgets and social media for both entertainment and education. When this limit is mutually agreed upon, parents must make extra efforts to respect these limits, and not assume unhindered access to gadgets for parents because of their authority and position in the family. Rules that apply to children should be reasonably applicable to the parents as well, for example, no gadgets during meals. Third, decide together what the correct course of action is for making amends every time someone flouts the generally agreed-upon use of social media and the internet. It helps to examine with children the statistics about the environmental cost of using generative AI and the high amount of energy and water the data centers use. When sensitive children learn about how every AI prompt causes an environmental impact, it is likely that they will reconsider their AI use.

Transparency

We have interacted with some parents who find it very difficult to accept that their teenage children are watching porn online. Here, it is critical to note that internet use among young children must be strictly monitored in order to protect them from inappropriate content and dangerous people. We should, however, also be ready to accept that as children mature, they will use these devices for intimate and personal purposes. To ensure transparency with children, discuss safe ways of using the internet with children. Introduce children to the idea of incognito windows, but also discuss with them the consequences of uploading private photos online, as any online repository and storage can be easily hacked. Help your children navigate away from violent porn, and discuss how watching aggression and violence can create unrealistic expectations in their minds and eventually be detrimental to their relationships.

Many Indian parents snoop on their teenage children's phones and call them out for a text they sent, a message they wrote, or the photos they shared on their Instagram. If parents use an authoritative approach to control their children's social media use, children will find more discreet ways of hiding their online life from their parents. Remember, they are not obliged to share their passwords with you, and there are umpteen ways of holding multiple secret accounts on the internet. So, if we want to protect our children from possible dangers and threats, we must try to develop a rapport with our children, to understand their world, which has changed from when we were their age, and to make them trust us, so that they are ready to share their online spaces and activities with us.

Digital and AI Literacy

Digital literacy is the active process of equipping children and young people with information about the threats involved in using digital media, especially the internet and social media. For Gen Alpha, and their parents, AI literacy is equally important. Critical AI literacy means not only learning various AI tools for productivity and fun, but also learning about their personal, societal, and ethical implications. We also familiarize children with resources for avoiding, challenging, and reporting harmful content. Before allowing children to access social media, parents must hold a detailed discussion with them related to all the possible perils of using social media uncritically. Parents can use different examples to discuss the consequences of cyberbullying, online sexual abuse, identity fraud, and other cyberthreats. A strategy to create awareness among children around cyberbullying and other dangers is to hold co-viewing sessions, where parents and children can watch documentaries, shows, and stories about indiscriminate use of the internet, social media use, and its dangers. The intention is not to scare them, but to prepare them well. For children above the age of 12 years, shows can be a good starting point to initiate discussions around bullying, sexual abuse, exploitation, threats, and privacy topics.

Strategies for Fighting Cyberbullying and Online Abuse

- Teach them to never post or say anything on the internet that they would not want the whole world—including you—to read.
- Talk to them about reaching out to an adult at the first sign of a threat. Do not take for granted that your child will be forthcoming.
- Chill! Kids refuse to confide in their parents because they're scared that if they find out about cyberbullying, they will take away their internet or mobile phone.
- Teach your children that what goes on online is everyone's business. Let them know that action must be taken when cyberbullying is encountered. Not reporting it is tantamount to approving it.

- Encourage kids to speak out against bullying when they see it. Popular sites like Facebook and YouTube provide tools for reporting inappropriate content, and the "comments" features associated with individual pages can provide opportunities for witnesses to speak out.
- Do not fight back. A lot of times bullies are looking to get a rise out of the kids they are targeting, and fighting back just gives them what they want.
- Save the evidence. Tell your children to make sure they have a record of what happened if somebody is mean to them online. If it is something that was sent directly to them, make sure they save it. If it's something that can be deleted (a tweet, a status update, etc.), have them take a screenshot.
- Talk to somebody. Make sure that your kids know that they can always come to you or another trusted adult if they are in trouble. If there's no one they can talk to offline, remind them that they can reach out to helplines and talk to one of their trained counselors. It is helpful to search and keep a note of helplines that you find trustworthy.
- Remember to remind them that it is not their fault if they are being cyberbullied. Nothing they do makes it okay for people to be mean to them, and nothing about them justifies people being mean to them.

It is extremely crucial to remind your children of the consequences of bullying others in order to ensure that they do not become the perpetrators. Monitor your children's online activities to make sure they are not involved in any online fraud, identity theft, or other criminal activities.

As we are examining online activities and engagement of children, we must also pay attention to the narratives of online games that children play. Sometimes, these online games are extremely violent and aggressive. Such games encourage the use of online abuse and normalize discursive violence. Also, some games are not age appropriate. It is, therefore, necessary that families create a healthy media diet and follow it.

Designing the Family Media Diet

As parents, we take great care in planning healthy meals for our children. A healthy media diet is just as important. Parents and children can create a timetable delineating their digital use, so that each member of the house is allowed to access gadgets, technologies, or social media for a limited amount of time. Similar discipline and transparency is required for family AI use as well. It is also crucial to ponder the concept of a "sacred space," which is devoid of any and every technological intrusion. This sacred space, such as the dinner table, the library, or the bedroom, should ideally allow family members to engage with each other in the complete absence of any technological mediation. For instance, parents choose to leave their phones at home when they are taking their children to parks, hotels, or movie theaters.

A rich family media diet must include a good mix of co-viewing and personal viewing practices. Co-viewing strategies are very effective in helping children interpret media messages and online activities. Even if it is not possible to commit to a co-viewing practice, parents can ask their children about what they watch and read. It is equally helpful when parents enroll themselves in supportive peer groups and subscribe to newsletters and mailing lists to receive suggestions about good media products that are fun, enriching, and stimulating for their families. Co-creating creative projects using technology—such as greeting cards, festive messages, memory books, and travel albums—also helps to initiate conversations around technology and many other topics, but it is equally important to plan non-media activities for the family. Many times, children turn to their gadgets because of boredom, loneliness, and a lack of other interesting activities.

Questions Parents Can Ask to Monitor their Children's Media Choices and Interpretive Skills

- Tell me what happened in the show.
- What did the characters do?
- Do you agree with what the characters did? Why, or why not?
- What did the characters talk about?
- How did you feel watching the show? Why?
- What was your favorite part? Why?
- What part did you not like? Why?
- What questions do you have? (e.g., meaning of words, actions of characters, etc.)
- What is the most fascinating part of the game you are playing?
- What strategies have you developed for cracking different game levels or winning?

Of course, kids should not feel that they are being interrogated or tested every time they watch something new! Creating a family's media diet includes assessing three things: How much time we are spending on media technologies; Why we are using media technologies, i.e., the purpose; and How we can include diversity in the media we are consuming as a family—the genre, content, issue, origin, and other topics.

The time criterion decides the amount of time a family spends on media. It is recommended that young people should not spend more than two hours per day on digital media. Creating shared ground rules for how long children and parents can use digital media per day is a democratic process, because it involves discussions and shared meaning-making. Another strategy is to block out a large part of the day for "no digital media" use. For instance, in many families, no one is allowed to use their phones and laptops before heading out for work and after coming back home. Some people also install applications that set a daily usage limit for various social media platforms to no more than two hours per day. Second, in today's technologized world, most of us rely on our gadgets for work and education. Dividing the time spent on gadgets for work and leisure purposes can help us save the time we waste scrolling through others' profiles and watching memes for hours at a stretch, or substitute playing video games for going out to playgrounds or parks. Finally, analyzing and actively selecting meaningful content to further the growth and well-being of our children through media consumption is a very important step. The media provide avenues for discussing social issues, unburdening ourselves through humor, or feeling inspired and energized to work more efficiently the next day. Media experiences can be both critical and grounding in nature. We can choose to watch, read, and listen to media designed to challenge our thought processes and force us out of our complacency toward ourselves and our communities. Of course, we use media to relax, to laugh, to escape into fantasy worlds, and to bond with other family members over shared programs. There are thankfully many movies, shows, podcasts, and OTT content that combine fun with sensitivity. Some media narratives reinforce the status quo in societies and reify discrimination. If we are not vigilant, we may fall prey to media narratives that are produced only to generate revenue, without any regard for the mental well-being of the viewers. Many shows on television, for instance, perpetuate patriarchal and misogynistic behavior, and this can be detrimental to the growth and progress of our communities. Our minds are like our bodies: we must be very careful of what we put in them.

Build a family media plan that grows with your child. Partner with schools, so policies explicitly cover image-based abuse and AI-manipulated media, and so students are graded for process as well as product, documenting sources, noting AI use, and practicing reporting pathways. The stance to carry forward is simple and steady: Gen Alpha's world is not going offline, so our job is to raise platform-literate, AI-aware kids who know how to spot risk, exit early, ask for help, and repair when harm occurs. Conscious parenting makes that possible by turning worry into routines, values into choices a child can name, and digital spaces into places where judgment, agency, and care stay at the center.

Ultimately, Gen Alpha will require some help from parents in unplugging from technology and learning to build relationships in real, and not just virtual, world. Creating shared and meaningful experiences with and without technology will go a long way in creating family memories that the children will cherish forever.

7 Gen Alpha as Citizens of the World

Children as Citizens of the World

Let's start with what children can already see and experience: a history project that pairs a classroom in Pune with one in Pretoria; a cousin who studies in Singapore but celebrates Diwali on video at 6 a.m.; a weekend robotics meet where coaches speak Hindi, Tamil, Marathi—and Spanish; a playlist that moves from K-pop to Punjabi pop without apology. This isn't a brochure for globalization; it is the texture of daily life. Indian schools using international curricula, multinational teams in local offices, student exchanges and summer institutes, families traveling more often, global brands on the high street, and online communities that shrink distance—all of it means our children are growing up with constant exposure to people whose languages, histories, and hopes do not mirror their own. The educational task is not to tack on a "global day," but to help children build the dispositions and skills to move from local comfort to global competence: curiosity that asks good questions, humility that expects to learn, empathy that stretches across difference, and judgment that holds firm to fairness when norms collide.

A global citizen, then, is not a child who collects stamps or accents; it is a child who understands that rights and responsibilities do not stop at the city border, who can hold two truths at once—deep roots and open doors. They read news beyond one country and notice whose stories are missing. They can compare what the same problem—air pollution, water scarcity, migration, online safety—looks like in different places, and how solutions travel or fail. They practice intercultural communication, which means more than "speaking English" or ordering sushi; it means listening for context, recognizing power differences, and adjusting with respect. They learn that global also means planetary: climate, biodiversity, and public health are shared fates. And because much of life now happens online, they treat digital citizenship as part of global citizenship—verifying sources across borders, resisting disinformation, protecting privacy, and participating in communities that include people they may never meet in-person.

To get there, we have to clear up a few myths. First, consumption is not citizenship. Enjoying global cuisine, streaming international shows, adopting

DOI: 10.4324/9781003590040-7

Western fashion, or traveling frequently does not automatically build global empathy; it can just as easily become lifestyle tourism. Second, being global does not require being rootless. The best global citizens tend to be well-rooted—grounded in their own languages, literatures, and rituals—because secure identity makes space for genuine curiosity, rather than defensive comparison. Third, sending a child to an international school with foreign languages and a long co-curricular list is not a guarantee. Without intentional teaching about history, power, and equity, such privileges can harden bubbles, instead of opening minds. And performative add-ons don't fix this: learning a language without learning the people's history; logging "charity hours" only to satisfy a school requirement; going on an exchange trip, while refusing to host a student from another background at home—these are signals without substance. The test is reciprocity and respect: Do we learn with others, not just about them? Do we offer hospitality as readily as we accept it? Do we honor our own traditions, while making room for someone else's?

Before we can introduce our children to the idea of "citizens of the world," we must first define what it means to be a global citizen. First, being a global citizen does not mean we stop being the citizens of our country or lose all attachment to our city, state, and local culture. We can be local, national, and global citizens at the same time. At the heart of Global Citizenship is the concept of shared human experience, which transcends geographical, cultural, and other barriers. Global citizenship has the following distinct features:

- Transcultural awareness: We have been exploring the concept of transcultural citizenship for more than a decade now. We argue that, though people are now globally connected through the internet and digital networks, they are still rooted in their local realities. Transcultural awareness is a very critical feature of globally oriented children and emphasizes that young people experience the world, different people, regions, countries, and communities culturally and relationally. For instance, students who participate in global exchange programs develop close bonds with individuals from other countries and they learn about different cultures and communities in and through their interpersonal interactions with their global partners. At the same time, students who have never traveled abroad due to a lack of resources can also forge such ties and friendships through online communities or even through reading books from across the world. Books are the cheapest way to get a glimpse of the world.

We also emphasize the importance of the local in today's globalized world, and that is the second component of global citizenship:

- Rootedness in local realities: Globally oriented people operate from within their local, everyday realities. For instance, when a young person from India writes blogs on social issues related to the environment or gender equity for international and global platforms, they will provide examples

and instances based on what they observe in their cities and communities. At the same time, our local realities are changing every day because of global influences. For instance, the uproar around Black Lives Matter in May of 2020 in international media encouraged many people in India to question colorism and caste-based discrimination in their own societies. As a result of such questioning, young people in India compelled a fairness cream to rebrand itself in order to challenge the practice of colorism. Though this is a very small step, it exemplifies how global issues influence our local experiences. To be globally oriented, young people must relate to their local communities and then form links globally. If this does not happen, they might feel rootless and lost.
- Technological and safety skills: The internet and digital networks can help us develop a multicultural perspective. We learn to respect and understand different cultures. This certainly does not mean that all people everywhere are the same. The internet allows children to experience the world and the differences inherent in human societies firsthand. Tell us, how else can you do this at such a low cost without traveling abroad? If we equip our children, or rather support them to equip themselves, with the necessary technological skills and safety measures, children can use online spaces as arenas of learning. It helps them reach places and people beyond their physical reach, meet people with very different ideologies, and learn how to engage with these differences.
- Adaptability: The rate of change these days is so rapid that all of us must learn to accept and adapt to change. Everything around us and our children is changing dramatically—from modes of teaching and learning, to ways of communicating and connecting, to systems of trade and commerce, to jobs, and places to look for a life partner.

How do the above features translate as practice in families and schools?

- Pair every foreign language with place, history, and literature, so words carry people, not just grammar. When a child studies French, let them meet Senegalese and Québécois voices, not only Parisians.
- When a class builds a service project, co-design it with community partners, and measure dignity, not just hours.
- Rotate leadership, so all children learn to both speak and listen across differences.
- Bring in role models whose lives cross the false divides—an Indian conservationist working with Kenyan rangers; a nurse who codes; a queer entrepreneur building inclusive workplaces.
- Create a global news habit: one Indian outlet, one regional outlet from another part of the world, and one issue-focused source; discuss how headlines frame the same event differently.
- Online, help children join supportive communities—book exchanges, open-source coding groups, global Model UNs, citizen science projects—where

contribution matters more than popularity. Teach them to introduce themselves clearly, to ask for consent before sharing photos or names, and to disagree without dehumanizing, as members of diverse communities.

Finally, help children connect scales—from local to global and back again. A river clean-up is local; the science of watersheds and climate makes it global. A class pen-pal project is local; learning why a friend's school closes during heat-waves makes it global. Hosting an exchange student is local; noticing which foods comfort them far from home—and asking what comforts you when you travel—teaches reciprocity that global conferences rarely can. By trying action to make context, we raise children who see beyond borders and discrimination of caste, class, color, and creed, without discarding their own culture. The goal is not to manufacture "citizens of nowhere," but to nurture citizens who carry their home lightly and their responsibilities widely, remaining curious, grounded, critical, kind. When a child can greet difference without fear, spot common cause across oceans, form supportive communities online and off, contribute to movements with care, and keep themselves and others safe in an interconnected world, "global citizen" stops being a slogan and becomes a way of moving through the world that is worthy of the name.

Using Social Media Purposefully

Young people should certainly have the freedom to use social media for fun, leisure, friendship, and entertainment, but they can extend their social media use to include practices that allow them to make civic contributions through discussions, online activism, and conversations. Such a choice should not be forced on young people, but we should at least expose them to the possibilities.

Let's first understand what it means for young people to be civically active. A civic-minded person has three core characteristics:

1. They try to identify and examine the problems in the communities.
2. They try to take responsibility for their actions in relation to society. Some questions to consider may include: Am I littering in the streets? Am I encouraging bullying or any form of harassment in my classrooms and playgrounds? Am I not being fair to someone because of my bias?
3. They try to make their communities better through discussions, activism, or volunteering.

If our children want to make meaningful connections over the internet, it is important that we educate them to use their social media to create sensitive and well-meaning dialogues with others. Young people sometimes use the anonymity and distance embedded in social media to abuse, bully, and threaten others. We must look at our social media as the new public forum, where people should be encouraged to hold deliberations and conversations of public interest.

Echo Chambers on Social Media

Here, a critical point to consider is how the network algorithms of social media platforms limit us within echo chambers. Algorithmic studies suggest that interactions of individuals on their social media are determined by their peer networks, i.e., who are their friends, what kinds of posts do they like and share, who do they engage with on a regular basis through their social media platforms, and so on. Young people need critical adult guidance on how to hold meaningful one-to-one conversations online with those who lie outside our echo chambers, i.e., those who have different opinions and ideologies. In the absence of such guidance, young individuals will continue to judge, stereotype, and bully others based on their life experiences. This can reinforce negative stereotypes and biases about the other. Parents and educators can guide young people out of their echo chambers and help them build inclusive and truly global social media networks and associations.

Countries have realized that our digitally connected world is sustained by interdependence and mutual respect for differences. As parents and teachers, it is our responsibility to nurture children as citizens of the world who are not fearful or anxious of differences, but meet them with curiosity and interest. Digital platforms and networks, our social media platforms, and the internet have afforded us innumerable opportunities to help our children experience the multicultural fabric of the world from their homes and schools.

As global citizens, children can:

- Form global friendships
- Learn about different countries and their cultures, religions, environments, and politics
- Represent their local culture, realities, and issues to the world
- Seek collaboration over issues of common interest
- Join communities of interest
- Raise funds for local and global causes
- Become global empaths

Can we think of ways in which children can use the media and technology to connect beyond the classrooms, beyond local and national borders, and learn to embrace differences? What unique challenges would Gen Alpha face in the process?

Connecting Beyond Borders and Differences

Young people from around the world have similar civic interests and want to collaborate with others in order to think about ways to change the world. For instance, many young bloggers from different countries are connected to the issue of environmental conservation. They discuss ways in which they could protect their environment and write/sign petitions demanding that governments and corporations adopt more environmentally friendly policies. Though these children have different lifestyles, experiences, cultures, and societies, the internet allows them to identify points of similarity with others and to bridge those differences through collective teamwork. During our conversations, a young blogger from Sri Lanka explained,

> The blogging internship program that I participated in has young people from Japan, India, New York, and many other places across the globe. It helps the young bloggers to share and exchange ideas, interact with issues that seem very distant, only to realize that such problems are very much a concern in their local environments as well. We can identify how the problems take different forms, as and when the context and culture change.

As is evident, internet networks and platforms help young people find common connections with others and use those similarities in interests to bridge cultural gaps.

To forge global connections, young people need adult guidance and encouragement. Very few children use the potential of internet for creative purposes on their own. Many are not aware of such opportunities, and so it is the responsibility of parents and educators to introduce children to creative, communicative, and global possibilities over the internet. Instead of spending endless hours on social media, scrolling through other people's feeds, children can be encouraged to use their time to blog about issues that interest them. The infrastructure of social media and the internet is revolutionary because it enables connections, creations, and networking across countries and platforms at affordable rates. Also, the internet offers rich resources in mentorship, guidance, or training. YouTube has many tutorials on several topics- from gardening, cooking, solving math problems, coding, and dancing, to artwork, public speaking, rhetoric, and much more. Some of these platforms can also open up possibilities for spending quality parent–child time, and can lead children to being part of global communities which share the same interests

AI, when used ethically and with discretion, can also be an aid in cultivating global sensitivity. For example, AI offers unprecedented opportunities to practice a new language. AI offers Gen Alpha something earlier generations never had at scale: a low-stakes, always-available partner for real conversation in another language. A child can ask a chatbot to role-play a shopkeeper, a bus conductor, a soccer coach, or a museum guide and practice exactly the phrases they'll need next week—ordering snacks, asking directions, filing a library request—while the system adjusts speed, vocabulary, and accent to match the learner, and does not judge or embarrass the child for mistakes. Speech tools can listen and give gentle, specific feedback on pronunciation ("soften the 'r,' stress the second syllable"), then replay native examples from multiple regions, so children hear Spanish from Bogotá and Barcelona, Arabic from Cairo and Casablanca, English from Lagos and London. For shy learners, this is a gift: they can make mistakes privately, retry instantly, and build confidence before speaking to people face-to-face. For busy families, it means practice fits into everyday life—five minutes in a traffic jam, a quick dialogue before dinner, a caption explained during a soccer match—without waiting for the next class.

Because Gen Alpha lives in short, motivating loops, AI can gamify progress without dumbing it down: micro-missions ("order a meal under ⊠300"), daily streaks that reward consistency over cramming, and story quests that weave grammar into action. Crucially, these tools can be culture-rich, not culture-thin. With the right prompts, a learner can ask for idioms you'd actually hear in Nairobi or Naples, sample headlines from children's news in the target language, or script and record a mini-podcast with AI as producer—complete with vocabulary lists, context notes, and safer-search links for follow-up. Paired with translation and captioning, AI lets kids explore music, comics, and science videos made for peers abroad; language stops being a school subject and becomes a key that opens other people's everyday worlds.

This makes possible more honest global conversations about civic ideas. When Indian tweens swap voice notes with peers in the Gulf or North Africa about gender equity—or with classmates in Japan about climate preparedness—they discover that the same word can carry different weights. For one girl, "fighting for equality" might mean persuading her parents to let her finish secondary school; for another, it might mean campaigning for safer transit or equal pay. AI can support, not replace, these encounters: it can help kids prepare questions, unpack unfamiliar references, and translate replies accurately enough to keep the dialogue moving, while teachers and parents anchor the exchange in respect, consent, and context. That widening of perspective is what we mean by intersectional understanding—not agreeing on everything, but seeing how place, class, faith, policy, and family history shape what "freedom," "safety," or "rights" feel like in a real life.

As we transcend the geographical boundaries, "going global" should deepen, not dilute, the local. The best use of AI is to braid the two. Ask the tutor to compare festivals in Marathi and French, or to generate a neighborhood interview script in Hindi and Spanish, so a child can talk to a grandparent and a pen-pal about the same topic. Use translation to subtitle a student's short film about water shortages in their own neighborhood, then share it with partner classrooms abroad for feedback on solutions that worked elsewhere. Let AI draft a bilingual letter to the local ward office, but have children revise it together—choosing words that fit their street, their school, their city. In other words, AI should at once amplify roots and widen horizons—more voices, more access, more practice, and more empathy—so Gen Alpha learns new languages to connect with people, not to perform algorithms.

AI-powered language practice is not an end in itself; it is the on-ramp to real relationships and harder conversations. When a child can greet, question, and listen in someone else's tongue—even with the light support of captions or a tutor that suggests gentler phrasing, they are better equipped to join collaborations that matter; for example, co-writing a zine with peers abroad, debating a class resolution on transit safety, or trading voice notes about school rules and gender norms. The same tools that rehearse pronunciation can also help kids prepare respectful questions, unpack unfamiliar references, and translate replies well enough to keep meaning intact, so that dialogue moves beyond slogans into lived context. In that space, differences stop feeling like barriers and start becoming sources of insight—exactly the ground on which intersectional understanding grows. And because AI can weave local references into global exchanges, children learn to bring their own streets, families, and histories into the conversation, rather than leaving them at the door—setting up the next step: tying global empathy back to local action.

Engaging with others over creative pursuits or issues of civic importance can help our children identify ways in which they can understand themselves and the world better. For instance, young people from India discussing feminism and gender equity with others in the Arab countries may realize that everyone's definition of feminism is influenced by their lived realities. For a woman who has been raised in an extremely conservative and patriarchal society, arguing with her parents to allow her to complete her education is an act of challenging gender inequality. On the other hand, for a girl who belongs to a very progressive and feminist family, the right to education may not even be an issue of conflict or discussion. The process of developing sensitivity and empathy for other people and being considerate of their life struggles and realities is called intersectional understanding.

In the following section, we discuss how our global connections and understanding must be intrinsically tied to our local realities.

Understanding Your Place in the World: From Local to Global

The local is the centerpiece around which young people construct their global participation online. Let's look at the following example.

Scene I

Minakshi is a 16-year-old girl who lives in Delhi. She is enrolled in a school with students belonging to middle-class backgrounds. In the school, many students "slut-shame" students based on the clothes they wear, people they hang out with, or the boys they date. Minakshi has experienced this misogynistic behavior herself. She was slut-shamed for wearing a tube-top to a party at her friend's house.

When Minakshi discusses feminism and gender equity, she focuses primarily on how "women and girls are not allowed to wear what they want." She emphasizes, "Girls should wear what they want."

Scene II

Dina is a 16-year-old Muslim girl from Washington, DC. She knows Minakshi through a Facebook group where young girls discuss feminism, gender equity, girls in STEM (Science, Technology, Engineering, and Math), and other related issues. When Minakshi shared her experience related to clothing restrictions imposed on girls in her society, Dina shared a similar, yet very different experience. According to Dina, many of her friends and classmates often make her feel bad about wearing a hijab to classes and gatherings. Her school authorities also once thought about mandating a "no hijab in schools" rule. She is very offended that people continue to dictate how girls should dress or what clothes they should wear.

As is evident in both cases, even while discussing issues of global importance, such as feminism, gender equity, and women's safety, people choose to draw from their local life experiences. Through these global connections and communication, these young people develop ways to communicate their local experiences in ways that are relatable to a global audience.

This process, where young people demonstrate an awareness about the world, while making sense of and articulating their local realities, is called living globally. The most powerful case in point is examples of child climate activists from India who are collaborating with child activists from other countries to compel their respective governments to pass climate change laws. They discusses issues related to climate change and conservation, drawing from their local experiences of living in India. In their blogs, conversations, and speeches online, they discuss the local realities of climate degradation and tie it neatly to the global issue of climate change and global warming. Child activists are using local issues to draw attention to a global cause and to highlight how many of these societal issues may manifest in different forms locally, but will influence the entire world in these highly connected and globalized times.

In the following section, we suggest some online strategies our children might want to try to use in their social media spaces in order to generate meaningful dialogues around critical civic issues.

Online Strategies for Building Civic-Global Communities

Strategy I: Developing Online Production Skills

Social media platforms can be used to produce and circulate multimedia content to promote specific civic issues. Social media today use text, videos, images, animation, and sound. If we must encourage our children to use social media to develop their creative and production skills, then we must familiarize ourselves with the basic content creation principles of each platform.

Content on X is known for its brevity and precision. It is like précis writing skills. The aim is to create short and impactful passages discussing a particular issue.

Instagram is a photo-sharing platform which exploits the potential of the visual. To use Instagram effectively, young people must learn how to microblog using photos. The photos become the centerpiece around which the narrative is created.

Facebook relies more on interactions among people in the form of comments, responses, and messages shared in relation to any given post. Young people can be encouraged to follow pages and organizations where they are prompted to express their opinions on important civic issues. It is helpful for parents and children to look for appropriate online communities or websites together and to identify those where the children can participate in global issues and share their views. YouTube is a wonderful resource for young, budding technologists and artists who wish to share their content with people. Children who want to invite constructive criticism on their talents and work can submit their videos to various channels online for publication.

There are free and simple apps and software available to assist us with production, and it is great if our children want to learn to use them. While they are encouraged to do this, it is extremely important to remind them to use these channels in ways that keep them safe and unharmed.

Strategy II: Apply for Online Youth Development Programs and Join Online Youth Forums

When creating content for online audiences, it is important to understand the demands and needs of online communities. For instance, according to many content creators, online videos should not be anything longer than one minute because viewers start losing interest. They should also have a compelling storyline. This implies that young people require guidance and mentorship. Many organizations working with youth provide this kind of training. Some have fellowship training programs, where young people are encouraged to collaborate with global partners and co-create blog posts. These blog posts are then edited by senior bloggers to help children understand how they should address the needs of their global online audience. Some offer volunteering opportunities, where children can learn many skills. New programs keep emerging and, again, looking for them is a good way to spend time together.

Strategy III: Develop a Powerful and Ethical Public Voice

In times where the use of abuse and foul language is the new cool, it is important to emphasize the role of civil language and ethics to invite greater discussion and participation. Some of the most important insights we have gathered through our discussions with scholars, teachers, and parents over the years involve using sensitive language and focusing on the "similarities" among people, rather than magnifying the differences. It is very important to understand our differences and they are real; but very often, people find that there are more similarities in them than differences! Some crucial questions we can ask ourselves while engaging in online conversations with people from different socio-cultural, economic, and political backgrounds include:

- Am I treating the other person as I would like to be treated myself? Equally important, am I treating the other person the way they want to be treated?
- Am I being kind to other people, or am I trying to provoke them?
- Am I trying to understand the other person's situation, or am I trying to prove myself?
- Can I use logic, facts, and non-controversial statements to emphasize my point?
- Is my way of communicating with the other confrontational, or am I trying to address the issue at hand with patience and civic discipline?
- Do I resort to name calling, abuse, and using derogatory language when I think my point is being invalidated?
- Do I accept the gaps in my knowledge and attempt to learn from these discussions?
- How do I protect myself from online abuse in cases of heated discussion with others, without resorting to violent techniques?

Though social media provide a lot of opportunities, they also present threats and dangers. Critical social media use involves both harnessing its potential and avoiding its dangers. In earlier chapters, we discussed several strategies for safe social media and technology use. These strategies are helpful when Gen Alpha is heavily dependent on the internet and AI for building global relationships.

Of course, as Gen Alpha grows up, they will be exposed to many new technologies, platforms, and devices. Global issues may change in priorities. Relations between countries and cultures might change. The foundational skills discussed in this chapter, however, will stand Gen Alpha in good stead when they engage with the world as global citizens.

For Product Safety Concerns and Information please contact our EU representative GPSR@taylorandfrancis.com Taylor & Francis Verlag GmbH, Kaufingerstraße 24, 80331 München, Germany

Printed and bound by CPI Group (UK) Ltd, Croydon, CR0 4YY
20/04/2026
02093445-0014